The Complete Low Sodium Cookbook

- Lose the Salt but not the Flavor: Quickly and Low Budget Recipes for Boost Your Health Helping You Managing Your Kidney Disease -

[Simona Malcom]

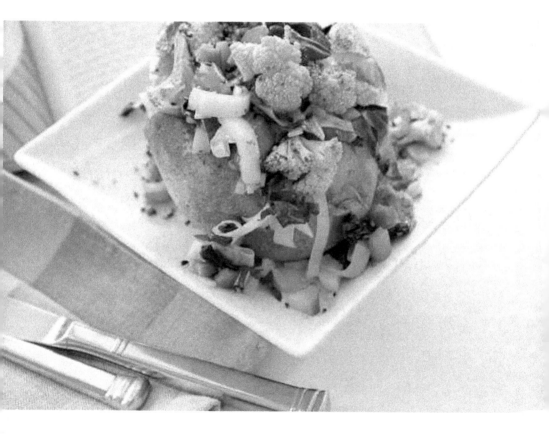

Table Of Contents

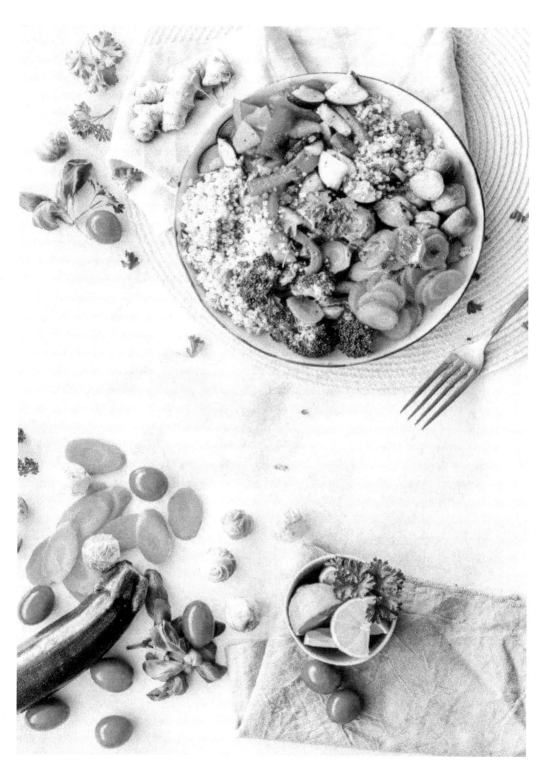

The following Book is reproduced below with the goal of providing information that is as accurate and reliable as possible. Regardless, purchasing this Book can be seen as consent to the fact that both the publisher and the author of this book are in no way experts on the topics discussed within and that any recommendations or suggestions that are made herein are for entertainment purposes only. Professionals should be consulted as needed prior to undertaking any of the action endorsed herein.

This declaration is deemed fair and valid by both the American Bar Association and the Committee of Publishers Association and is legally binding throughout the United States.

Furthermore, the transmission, duplication, or reproduction of any of the following work including specific information will be considered an illegal act irrespective of if it is done electronically or in print. This extends to creating a secondary or tertiary copy of the work or a recorded copy and is only allowed with the express written consent from the Publisher. All additional right reserved.

The information in the following pages is broadly considered a truthful and accurate account of facts and as such, any inattention, use, or misuse of the information in question by the reader will render any resulting actions solely under their purview. There are no scenarios in which the publisher or the original author of this work can be in any fashion deemed liable for any hardship or damages that may befall them after undertaking information described herein.

Additionally, the information in the following pages is intended only for informational purposes and should thus be thought of as universal. As befitting its nature, it is presented without assurance regarding its prolonged validity or interim quality. Trademarks that are mentioned are done without written consent and can in no way be considered an endorsement from the trademark holder.

CHAPTER 1: The Renal Diet

The Benefits of Renal diet

If you have been diagnosed with kidney dysfunction, a proper diet is necessary for controlling the amount of toxic waste in the bloodstream. When toxic waste piles up in the system along with increased fluid, chronic inflammation occurs, and we have a much higher chance of developing cardiovascular, bone, metabolic, or other health issues.

Since your kidneys can't fully get rid of the waste on their own, which comes from food and drinks, probably the only natural way to help our system is through this diet.

A renal diet is especially useful during the first stages of kidney dysfunction and leads to the following benefits:

● Prevents excess fluid and waste build-up

● prevents the progression of renal dysfunction stages

● Decreases the likelihood of developing other chronic health problems, e.g., heart disorders

● has a mild antioxidant function in the body, which keeps inflammation and inflammatory responses under control.

The benefits mentioned above are noticeable once the patient follows the diet for at least a month and then continuing it for longer periods to avoid the stage where dialysis is needed. The diet's strictness depends on the current stage of renal/kidney disease if, for example, if you are in the 3rd or 4th stage, you should follow a stricter diet and be attentive to the food, which is allowed or prohibited.

Nutrients You Need

Potassium

Potassium is a naturally occurring mineral found in nearly all foods in varying amounts. Our bodies need an amount of potassium to help with muscle activity as well as electrolyte balance and regulation of blood pressure. However, if potassium is in excess within the system and the kidneys can't expel it (due to renal disease), fluid retention and muscle spasms can occur.

Phosphorus

Phosphorus is a trace mineral found in a wide range of foods and especially dairy, meat, and eggs. It acts synergistically with calcium as well as Vitamin D to promote bone health. However, when there is damage in the kidneys, excess amounts of the mineral cannot be taken out, causing bone weakness.

Calories

When being on a renal diet, it is vital to give yourself the right number of calories to fuel your system. The exact number of calories you should consume daily depends on your age, gender, general health status, and stage of renal disease. In most cases, though, there are no strict limitations in the calorie intake, as long as you take them from proper sources that are low in sodium, potassium, and phosphorus. In general, doctors recommend a daily limit between 1800-2100 calories per day to keep weight within the normal range.

Protein

Protein is an essential nutrient that our systems need to develop and generate new connective tissue, e.g., muscles, even during injuries. Protein also helps stop bleeding and supports the immune system to fight infections. A healthy adult with no kidney disease would usually need 40-65 grams of protein per day.

However, in a renal diet, protein consumption is a tricky subject as too much or too little can cause problems. When metabolized by our systems, protein also creates waste, which is typically processed by the kidneys. However, when kidneys are damaged or underperforming, as in the case of kidney disease, that waste will stay in the system. This is why patients in more advanced CKD stages are advised to limit their protein consumption as well.

Fats

Our systems need fats and particularly good fats as a fuel source and for other metabolic cell functions. A diet high in bad or trans fats can significantly increase the chances of developing heart problems, which often occur with kidney disease. This is why most physicians advise their renal patients to follow a diet that contains a decent amount of good fats and a meager amount of Trans (processed) or saturated fat.

Sodium

Sodium is what our bodies need to regulate fluid and electrolyte balance. It also plays a role in normal cell division in the muscles and nervous system. However, in kidney disease, sodium can quickly spike at higher than normal levels, and the kidneys will be unable to expel it, causing fluid accumulation as a side-effect. Those who also suffer from heart problems as well should limit its consumption as it may raise blood pressure.

Carbohydrates

Carbs act as a major and quick fuel source for the body's cells. When we consume carbs, our systems turn them into glucose and then into energy for "feeding" our body cells. Carbs are generally not restricted in the renal diet. Still, some types of carbs contain dietary fiber as well, which helps regulate normal colon function and protect blood vessels from damage.

Dietary Fiber

Fiber is an important element in our system that cannot be properly digested, but plays a key role in the regulation of our bowel movements and blood cell protection. The fiber in the renal diet is generally encouraged as it helps loosen up the stools, relieve constipation and bloating and protect from colon damage. However, many patients don't get enough amounts of dietary fiber per day, as many of them are high in potassium or phosphorus. Fortunately, there are some good dietary fiber sources for CKD patients that have lower amounts of these minerals compared to others.

Vitamins/Minerals

According to medical research, our systems need at least 13 vitamins and minerals to keep our cells fully active and healthy. However, patients with renal disease are more likely to be depleted by water-soluble vitamins like B-complex and Vitamin C as a result of limited fluid consumption. Therefore, supplementation with these vitamins, along with a renal diet program, should help cover any possible vitamin deficiencies. Supplementation of fat-soluble vitamins like vitamins A, K, and E may be avoided as they can quickly build up in the system and turn toxic.

Fluids

When you are in an advanced stage of renal disease, fluid can quickly build-up and lead to problems. While it is important to keep your system well hydrated, you should avoid minerals like potassium and sodium, which can trigger further fluid build-up and cause a host of other symptoms.

Nutrient You Need to Avoid

Salt or sodium is known for being one of the most important ingredients that the renal diet prohibits its use. This ingredient, although simple, can badly and strongly affect your body, especially the kidneys. Any excess of sodium can't be easily filtered because of the failing condition of the kidneys. A large build-up of sodium can cause catastrophic results on your body. Potassium and Phosphorus are also prohibited for kidney patients depending on the stage of kidney disease.

CHAPTER 2: Kidney disease

What is Kidney Disease?

A kidney disease diagnosis implies that the kidneys are either dysfunctional, under-functioning, or damaged and cannot filter out toxins and metabolic waste on their own. Our systems need our kidneys for a waste filtering process. However, when kidney damage occurs, the system is piled up with damaging waste that cannot expel through other means. As a result, inflammatory responses emerge, and you have a much higher chance of developing chronic and serious health disorders like diabetes or heart failure, which can even be fatal in extreme cases.

There are two main types of kidney disease, based on their cause and time duration:

• A sudden and unexpected kidney damage/acute kidney injury (AKI) as a result of an accident or surgery side effects, which usually lasts for a short period of time.

• Chronic and progressive kidney dysfunction (CKD). As its name suggests, this is a chronic condition with multiple progressive stages that lead ultimately to permanent kidney damage. There are approx. 5 stages of the disorder, and during the last and final stage, the patient will need dialysis or a kidney transplant to survive. This final stage is also known in the medical glossary as End-Stage-Renal Disease (ESRD).

There are higher than normal amounts of a certain protein called Arbutin in the urine during all kidney dysfunction stages, which can be confirmed by urine tests for diagnosing renal disease. This condition is known scientifically as Proteinuria. Doctors may also perform blood tests and/or image screening tests to pinpoint a problem with the kidneys and develop a diagnosis.

Causes of Kidney Disease?

There are many causes of kidney disease, including physical injury or disorders that can damage the kidneys, but the two leading causes of kidney disease are diabetes and high blood pressure. These underlying conditions also put people at risk for developing cardiovascular disease. Early treatment may not only slow down the progression of the disease, but also reduce your risk of developing heart disease or stroke.

Kidney disease can affect anyone at any age. African Americans, Hispanics, and American Indians are at increased risk for kidney failure because these groups have a greater prevalence of diabetes and high blood pressure.

Uncontrolled diabetes is the leading cause of kidney disease. Diabetes can damage the kidneys and cause them to fail.

The second leading cause of kidney disease is high blood pressure, also known as hypertension. One in three Americans is at risk for kidney disease because of hypertension. Although there is no cure for hypertension, certain medications, a low-sodium diet, and physical activity can lower blood pressure.

The kidneys help manage blood pressure, but when blood pressure is high, the heart has to work overtime at pumping blood. High blood pressure can damage the blood vessels in the kidneys, reducing their ability to work efficiently. When the force of blood flow is high, blood vessels start to stretch so the blood can flow more easily. The stretching and scarring weaken the blood vessels throughout the entire body, including the kidneys. When the kidneys' blood vessels are injured, they may not remove the waste and extra fluid from the body, creating a dangerous cycle because the extra fluid in the blood vessels can increase blood pressure even more.

Cardiovascular disease is the leading cause of death in the United States. When kidney disease occurs, that process can be affected, and the risk of developing heart disease becomes greater. Cardiovascular disease is an umbrella term used to describe conditions that may damage the heart and blood vessels, including coronary artery disease, heart attack, heart failure, atherosclerosis, and high blood pressure. Complications from a renal disease may develop and can lead to heart disease.

With diabetes, excess blood sugar remains in the bloodstream. The high blood sugar levels can damage the blood vessels in the kidneys and elsewhere in the body. And since high blood pressure is a complication from diabetes, the extra pressure can weaken the walls of the blood vessels, which can lead to a heart attack or stroke.

Other conditions, such as drug abuse and certain autoimmune diseases, can also cause injury to the kidneys. In fact, every drug we put into our body has to pass through the kidneys for filtration. If the drug is not taken following a healthcare provider's instructions, or if it is an illegal substance such as heroin, cocaine, or ecstasy, it can cause injury to the kidneys by raising the blood pressure, also increasing the risk of a stroke, heart failure, and even death.

An autoimmune disease is one in which the immune system, designed to protect the body from illness, sees the body as an invader and attacks its own systems, including the kidneys. Some forms of lupus, for example, attack the kidneys. Another autoimmune disease that can lead to kidney failure is Goodpasture syndrome, a group of conditions that affect the kidneys and the lungs. The damage to the kidneys from autoimmune diseases can lead to chronic kidney disease and kidney failure.

Symptoms of Kidney Disease?

Some people in the early stages of kidney disease may not even show any symptoms. If you suffer from diabetes or high blood pressure, it is important to manage it early on in order to protect your kidneys. Although kidney failure occurs over the course of many years, you may not show any signs until kidney disease or failure has occurred.

When the kidneys are damaged, wastes and toxins can build up in the body because the kidneys cannot filter them as effectively. Once this buildup begins, you may start to feel sick and experience some of the following symptoms:

- Anemia (low red blood cell count)

- Blood in urine

- Bone pain

- Difficulty concentrating

- Difficulty sleeping

- Dry and itchy skin

- Muscle cramps (especially in the legs)

- Nausea

- Poor appetite

- Swelling in feet and ankles

- Tiredness

- Weakness

- Weight loss

Fortunately, once treatment for kidney disease begins, especially if caught in the early stages, symptoms tend to lessen, and general health will begin to improve.

Diagnosis Tests

Besides identifying the symptoms of kidney disease, there are other better and more accurate ways to confirm the extent of loss of renal function. There are mainly two important diagnostic tests:

1. Urine Test

The urine test clearly states all the renal problems. The urine is the waste product of the kidney. When there is a loss of filtration or any hindrance to the kidneys, the urine sample will indicate it through the number of excretory products present in it. The severe stages of chronic disease show some amount of protein and blood in the urine. Do not rely on self-tests; visit an authentic clinic for these tests.

2. Blood Pressure and Blood Test

Another good way to check for renal disease is to test the blood and its composition. A high amount of creatinine and other waste products in the blood clearly indicates that the kidneys are not functioning properly. Blood pressure can also be indicative of renal disease. When the water balance in the body is disturbed, it may cause high blood pressure. Hypertension can both be the cause and symptom of kidney disease and, therefore, should be taken seriously.

Treatment

The best way to manage CKD is to be an active participant in your treatment program, regardless of your stage of renal disease. Proper treatment involves a combination of working with a healthcare team, adhering to a renal diet, and making healthy lifestyle decisions. These can all have a profoundly positive effect on your kidney disease— especially watching how you eat.

Working with Your Healthcare Team

When you have kidney disease, working in partnership with your healthcare team can be extremely important in your treatment program as well as being personally empowering. Regularly meeting with your physician or healthcare team can arm you with resources and information that help you make informed decisions regarding your treatment needs and provide you with a much-needed opportunity to vent, share information, get advice, and receive support in effectively managing this illness.

Adhering to a Renal Diet

The heart of this book is the renal diet. Sticking to this diet can make a huge difference in your health and vitality. Like any change, following the diet may not be easy at first. Important changes to your diet, particularly early on, can possibly prevent the need for dialysis. These changes include limiting salt, eating a low-protein diet, reducing fat intake, and getting enough calories if you need to lose weight. Be honest with yourself first and foremost—learn what you need, and consider your personal goals and obstacles. Start by making small changes. It is okay to have some slip-ups—we all do. With guidance and support, these small changes will become habits of your promising new lifestyle. In no time, you will begin taking control of your diet and health.

Making Healthy Lifestyle Decisions

Lifestyle choices play a crucial part in our health, especially when it comes to helping regulate kidney disease. Lifestyle choices such as allotting time for physical activity, getting enough sleep, managing weight, reducing stress, and limiting smoking and alcohol will help you take control of your overall health, making it easier to manage your kidney disease. Follow this simple formula: Keep toxins out of your body as much as you can, and build up your immune system with a good balance of exercise, relaxation, and sleep.

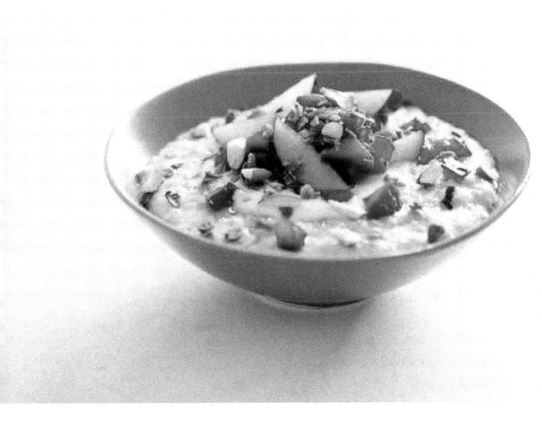

CHAPTER 3: **BREAKFAST**

Cheddar and Spinach Muffins

Prep:20 mins
Cook:35 mins
Servings:12

Ingredients

1 ½ cups all-purpose flour
1 egg
2 teaspoons baking powder
½ teaspoon salt
6 tablespoons butter, melted
½ teaspoon baking soda
1 cup whole milk
1 cup shredded Cheddar cheese
1 cup frozen chopped spinach - thawed, drained and squeezed dry

Directions

Preheat oven to 350 degrees F.
Lightly grease 12 cup muffin cups.
  2
Mix the flour, baking powder, baking soda, and salt together in a mixing bowl.
  3
Stir the melted butter, egg, milk, spinach, and Cheddar cheese together in a large mixing bowl until evenly blended. Slowly stir in the flour mixture to form a batter. Spoon 2 tablespoons into each muffin cup.
  4

Bake in preheated oven until a toothpick inserted into the center of a muffin comes out clean, about 30 minutes.

Nutrition

164 calories
protein 5.5g
carbohydrates 13.5g
fat 9.9g
cholesterol 42.3mg
sodium 349.3mg.

Eggplant Caprese

Prep:10 mins
Cook:10 mins
Servings:4

Ingredients

1 teaspoon grated fresh garlic
2 small purple eggplants, cut into 1/2-inch slices
½ teaspoon salt
1 tomato, sliced 1/8-inch thick
1 (8 ounce) package fresh mozzarella, thinly sliced
2 tablespoons olive oil
cooking spray
3 leaves fresh basil, cut into thin strips

Directions

Combine olive oil, garlic, and salt in a small bowl; set aside.
   2
Preheat an outdoor grill to 400 degrees F and lightly oil the grate.
   3
Put eggplant slices on the hot grill and cook for 3 to 4 minutes. Turn eggplant and brush with the oil mixture. Place 1 slice of tomato and 1 slice of mozzarella cheese on each eggplant piece. Close the lid and cook until cheese has melted, 3 to 4 minutes. Transfer to a plate and sprinkle with basil.

Nutrition

251 calories
protein 15.7g

carbohydrates 12.9g
fat 16.1g
cholesterol 35.8mg
sodium 642.8mg.

Easy Vegetable Pizza

Prep:25 mins
Additional:2 hrs
Servings:16

Ingredients

2 (8 ounce) packages refrigerated crescent rolls

1 cup sour cream

1 teaspoon dried dill weed

¼ teaspoon garlic salt

1 (8 ounce) package cream cheese, softened

1 (1 ounce) package ranch dressing mix

1 stalk celery, thinly sliced

½ cup halved and thinly-sliced radishes

1 red bell pepper, chopped

1 ½ cups fresh broccoli, chopped

1 carrot, grated

1 small onion, finely chopped

Directions

Preheat oven to 350 degrees F . Spray a jellyroll pan with non-stick cooking spray.

2

Pat crescent roll dough into a jellyroll pan. Let stand 5 minutes. Pierce with fork.

3

Bake for 10 minutes.

4

In a medium-sized mixing bowl, combine sour cream, cream cheese, dill weed, garlic salt and ranch dip mix. Spread this mixture on top of the cooled crust. Arrange the onion, carrot, celery, broccoli, radish, bell pepper and broccoli on top of the creamed mixture. Cover and let chill. Once chilled, cut it into squares and serve.

Nutrition

196 calories
protein 4.8g
carbohydrates 16g
fat 12.6g
cholesterol 35.7mg
sodium 358.6mg.

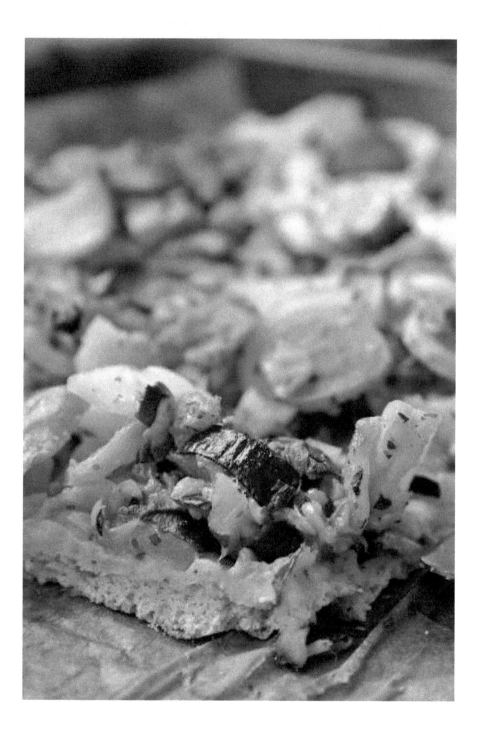

Fresh Shrimp Bruschetta

Prep:15 mins
Cook:5 mins
Additional:30 mins
Servings:12

Ingredients

½ pound chopped shrimp

1 (8 ounce) loaf French bread, sliced

2 cups mango, cut into small dice

½ cup lime juice

2 tablespoons honey, or more to taste

¼ cup chopped green onion

1 teaspoon cayenne pepper

1 (8 ounce) round Brie cheese, sliced

Directions

Stir the shrimp, mango, and green onion together in a bowl; set aside.
    2
Whisk the lime juice, honey, and cayenne pepper together in a separate bowl until blended, making sure to scrape along bottom of bowl as needed to incorporate honey; pour over the shrimp mixture. Cover with plastic wrap and refrigerate 30 minutes.
    3
Preheat an oven to 350 degrees F .
    4
Arrange the bread slices on a baking sheet. Top each bread slice with a slice of Brie cheese.
    5

Bake in the preheated oven until slightly browned and the Brie cheese is soft and melted, about 5 minutes. Top each slice with 1 tablespoon of the shrimp mixture to serve.

Nutrition

170 calories
protein 10.2g
carbohydrates 19.6g
fat 6g
cholesterol 47.7mg
sodium 271.2mg.

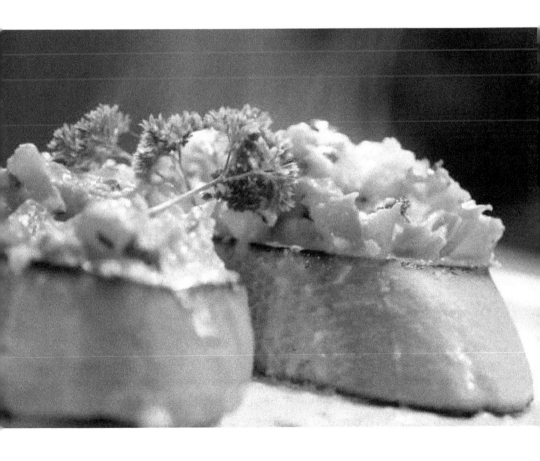

Master Vanilla Scones

Servings:8

Ingredients

2 cups all-purpose flour
⅓ cup sugar
¼ teaspoon baking soda
½ teaspoon salt
8 tablespoons unsalted butter, frozen
1 teaspoon baking powder
½ cup sour cream
1 large egg
½ cup raisins

Directions

Adjust oven rack to lower-middle position and preheat oven to 400 degrees.
2
In a medium bowl, mix flour, 1/3 cup sugar, baking powder, baking soda and salt. Grate butter into flour mixture on the large holes of a box grater; use your fingers to work in butter (mixture should resemble coarse meal), then stir in raisins.
3
In a small bowl, whisk sour cream and egg until smooth.
4
Using a fork, stir sour cream mixture into flour mixture until large dough clumps form. Use your hands to press the dough against the bowl into a ball. (The dough will be sticky in places, and there may not seem to be enough liquid at first, but as you press, the dough will come together.)
5

Place on a lightly floured surface and pat into a 7- to 8-inch circle about 3/4-inch thick. Sprinkle with remaining 1 tsp. of sugar. Use a sharp knife to cut into 8 triangles; place on a cookie sheet (preferably lined with parchment paper), about 1 inch apart. Bake until golden, about 17 minutes. Cool for 5 minutes and serve warm or at room temperature.

Nutrition

319 calories;
protein 4.9g;
carbohydrates 41.1g;
fat 15.5g;
cholesterol 60.1mg;
sodium 249.3mg.

Rustic Olive Bread

Prep:20 mins
Cook:45 mins
Additional:2 hrs 15 mins
Servings:24

Ingredients

2 ½ cups warm water (110 degrees F)

2 tablespoons active dry yeast

1 tablespoon salt

7 ½ cups bread flour

1 teaspoon molasses

1 cup kalamata olives, pitted and chopped

2 tablespoons chopped fresh rosemary

2 tablespoons olive oil

Directions

Place water, yeast, and molasses in a mixing bowl; stir to mix. Let stand for a few minutes until mixture is creamy and foamy.

2

Add olive oil and salt; mix. Add flour, about a cup at a time, until dough is too stiff to stir. Add olives and fresh herbs.

3

Turn dough out onto a lightly floured board. Knead, adding flour as needed to keep from being sticky, until smooth and elastic. Place in well oiled bowl, and turn to coat the dough surface with oil. Allow to rise until doubled in bulk, about an hour or so.

4

Punch the dough down, split into two pieces, and form into two round loaves. Place on greased baking sheet . Spray with cold water and sprinkle with sesame seeds if desired. Let loaves rise for 30 minutes.

5

Bake at 400 degrees F for 45 minutes.

Nutrition

186 calories
protein 5.7g;
carbohydrates 32.3g;
fat 3.6g;
sodium 383.9mg.

Cabbage Cakes

Prep:15 mins
Cook:15 mins
Servings:15

Ingredients

1 tablespoon olive oil
½ small head cabbage, cored and sliced thin
black pepper to taste
1 ⅓ cups plain yogurt
⅔ cup milk
1 onion, thinly sliced
¼ cup vegetable oil
2 eggs
1 onion, thinly sliced
2 cups flour
1 teaspoon baking soda
1 teaspoon butter
4 teaspoons baking powder

Directions

Heat the olive oil in a large skillet over medium heat. Stir in the
cabbage and onion; cook and stir until the vegetables are soft and
fragrant, about 10 minutes. Season with pepper, and set pan aside to
cool.
    2
Whisk together the yogurt, milk, vegetable oil, and eggs in a bowl until
evenly blended; set aside. Stir together the flour, baking powder, and
baking soda in a large bowl. Make a well in the center of the dry
Ingredients. Pour the wet mixture into the well, then stir until well

combined. Fold the cooled cabbage and onions into the pancake batter.

3

Heat a large skillet over medium heat, and butter or oil if necessary. Pour 1/4 cupfuls of batter onto the skillet, and cook until bubbles appear on the surface. Flip with a spatula, and cook until browned on the other side.

Nutrition

142 calories;
protein 4.5g;
carbohydrates 17.3g;
fat 6.2g;
cholesterol 27.7mg;
sodium 249.8mg.

Italian Panzanella Salad

Prep:30 mins
Cook:20 mins
Servings:8

Ingredients

6 cups day old Italian bread, torn into bite-size pieces
⅓ cup olive oil
3 cloves garlic, minced
¼ cup olive oil
salt and pepper to taste
2 tablespoons balsamic vinegar
¾ cup sliced red onion
10 basil leaves, shredded
4 medium ripe tomatoes, cut into wedges
½ cup pitted and halved green olives
1 cup fresh mozzarella, cut into bite-size pieces

Directions

Preheat oven to 400 degrees F .
   2
In a large bowl, toss bread with 1/3 cup olive oil, salt, pepper, and garlic. Lay bread on a baking sheet, and toast in the preheated oven until golden, about 10 minutes; allow to cool slightly.
   3
While the bread is in the oven, whisk together 1/4 cup of olive oil and balsamic vinegar. Gently toss together the bread, tomatoes, onion, basil, olives, and mozzarella cheese. Toss with the vinaigrette and let stand for 20 minutes before serving.

Nutrition

308 calories;
protein 6.6g;
carbohydrates 22.2g;
fat 21.7g;
cholesterol 11.8mg;
sodium 551.4mg.

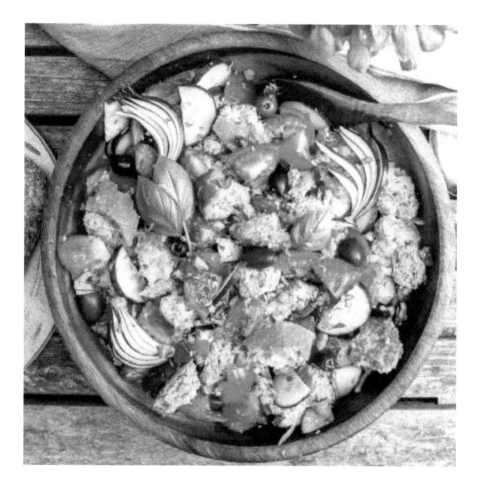

Yufka Pastry Pies

Prep:30 mins
Cook:50 mins
Additional:10 mins
Servings:12

Ingredients

2 cups frozen peas and carrots
1 cup sliced celery
⅔ cup butter
½ teaspoon onion powder
4 (9 inch) unbaked pie crusts
⅔ cup chopped onion
2 cups frozen green beans
1 teaspoon salt
1 teaspoon ground black pepper
½ teaspoon celery seed
½ teaspoon Italian seasoning
1 ¾ cups chicken broth
1 ⅓ cups milk
⅔ cup all-purpose flour
4 cups cubed cooked turkey meat - light and dark meat mixed

Directions

Preheat an oven to 425 degrees F .
   2
Place the peas and carrots, green beans, and celery into a saucepan;
cover with water, bring to a boil, and simmer over medium-low heat
until the celery is tender, about 8 minutes. Drain the vegetables in a
colander set in the sink, and set aside.
   3

Melt the butter in a saucepan over medium heat, and cook the onion until translucent, about 5 minutes. Stir in 2/3 cup of flour, salt, black pepper, celery seed, onion powder, and Italian seasoning; slowly whisk in the chicken broth and milk until the mixture comes to a simmer and thickens. Remove from heat; stir the cooked vegetables and turkey meat into the filling until well combined.

4

Fit 2 pie crusts into the bottom of 2 9-inch pie dishes. Spoon half the filling into each pie crust, then top each pie with another crust. Pinch and roll the top and bottom crusts together at the edge of each pie to seal, and cut several small slits into the top of the pies with a sharp knife to release steam.

5

Bake in the preheated oven until the crusts are golden brown and the filling is bubbly, 30 to 35 minutes. If the crusts are browning too quickly, cover the pies with aluminum foil after about 15 minutes. Cool for 10 minutes before serving.

Nutrition

539 calories;
protein 20.4g;
carbohydrates 39.5g;
fat 33.2g;
cholesterol 64.7mg;
sodium 650.7mg.

Creamy Radish Soup

Prep:15 mins
Cook:45 mins
Servings:6

Ingredients

2 tablespoons butter
1 large onion, diced
4 cups raw radish greens
4 cups chicken broth
⅓ cup heavy cream
5 radishes, sliced
2 medium potatoes, sliced

Directions

Melt butter in a large saucepan over medium heat. Stir in the onion, and saute until tender. Mix in the potatoes and radish greens, coating them with the butter. Pour in chicken broth. Bring the mixture to a boil. Reduce heat, and simmer 30 minutes.

2

Allow the soup mixture to cool slightly, and transfer to a blender. Blend until smooth.

3

Return the mixture to the saucepan. Mix in the heavy cream. Cook and stir until well blended. Serve with radish slices.

Nutrition

166 calories; protein 3.8g; carbohydrates 17.9g; fat 9.3g; cholesterol 31.6mg; sodium 688.1mg.

Chia Bars

Prep:15 mins
Cook:30 mins
Additional:8 hrs 10 mins
Servings:24

Ingredients

4 cups water, divided
2 teaspoons salt
2 cups chopped almonds
cooking spray
3 cups all-purpose flour
⅔ cup chocolate chips
⅔ cup olive oil
1 pinch salt
⅔ cup chia seeds
½ cup powdered peanut butter (such as PB2®)
1 tablespoon ground cinnamon
2 teaspoons vanilla extract
½ cup honey

Directions

Combine 2 cup water, almonds, and 1 pinch salt together in a bowl; let sit for 8 hours to overnight. Drain and rinse 2 times.
    2
Blend drained almonds and 2 cups water together in a blender until smooth, about 2 minutes. Transfer to a large bowl.
    3
Preheat oven to 350 degrees F (175 degrees C). Spray an 11x15-inch baking dish with cooking spray.
    4

Mix flour, chocolate chips, olive oil, chia seeds, honey, powdered peanut butter, cinnamon, vanilla extract, and 2 teaspoons salt into almond mixture until dough is evenly combined. Transfer dough to the prepared baking dish, leveling dough with a fork or spatula.

    5

Bake in the preheated oven until cooked through and lightly browned, 35 - 45 minutes. Allow to cool for 10 minutes before cutting into bars.

Nutrition

248 calories;
protein 5.5g;
carbohydrates 25.8g;
fat 14.8g;
sodium 215.1mg.

Shrimp Omelet

Prep:30 mins
Cook:25 mins
Servings:3

Ingredients

¼ cup chicken broth
1 (6 ounce) can salad shrimp
1 tablespoon Dijon mustard
2 tablespoons butter
1 (6 ounce) can crab
¼ cup heavy cream

Sauce:
¼ cup heavy cream
1 cup shredded Cheddar cheese
1 dash nutmeg
Salt and pepper to taste
1 teaspoon Dijon mustard

Omelets:
4 eggs, beaten
Salt and pepper to taste
¼ cup heavy cream

Directions

Prepare the filling by stirring Dijon mustard into chicken broth in a saucepan until dissolved. Bring to a simmer over medium-high heat, then add 1/4 cup cream and 2 tablespoons butter. Reduce heat to medium, and simmer until reduced by half, then stir in crab and shrimp; keep warm over low heat.

2

Prepare the sauce by warming 1/4 cup cream, and 1 teaspoon mustard over medium heat. Once hot, whisk in the shredded cheese, then season to taste with nutmeg, salt, and pepper. Keep warm over low heat.

3

Whisk eggs, 1/4 cup cream, salt, and pepper together until smooth. Heat an 8-inch non-stick skillet over medium heat, and lightly oil with cooking spray. Pour 1/4 cup of the egg mixture into hot pan, and swirl to make a thin, even layer of egg. Cook until firmed, then flip and cook for a few seconds more to firm the other side.

4

To prepare omelets, spoon some of the seafood filling into the lower half of each omelet. Roll up into a cylinder. Serve 2 per person bathed with Cheddar sauce.

Nutrition

652 calories;
protein 43.5g;
carbohydrates 4.8g;
fat 50.7g;
cholesterol 536.1mg;
sodium 852.2mg.

Aragula Salad with Shaved Parmesan

Prep:15 mins
Servings:4

Ingredients

4 cups young arugula leaves, rinsed and dried
1 tablespoon rice vinegar
1 cup cherry tomatoes, halved
¼ cup pine nuts
1 large avocado - peeled, pitted and sliced
2 tablespoons grapeseed oil
freshly ground black pepper to taste
¼ cup grated Parmesan cheese
salt to taste

Directions

In a large plastic bowl with a lid, combine arugula, cherry tomatoes, pine nuts, oil, vinegar, and Parmesan cheese. Season with salt and pepper to taste. Cover, and shake to mix.
    2
Divide salad onto plates, and top with slices of avocado.

Nutrition

257 calories;
protein 6.2g;
carbohydrates 10g;
fat 23.2g;
cholesterol 4.4mg;
sodium 381.3mg.

Happy Cauliflower Pancake

Prep:15 mins
Cook:36 mins
Servings:12

Ingredients

1 tablespoon coconut oil
1 teaspoon olive oil
2 cups grated cauliflower
¼ cup egg whites
1 clove garlic, minced
1 cup 1% cottage cheese, drained
2 tablespoons finely chopped onion
1 tablespoon hot pepper sauce
1 teaspoon dried oregano
¼ teaspoon garlic powder
2 teaspoons dried parsley

Directions

Preheat the oven to 350 degrees F . Grease a 12-cup muffin tin with coconut oil.

2

Heat olive oil in a skillet over medium heat. Add cauliflower, onion, and garlic. Cook and stir until cauliflower is slightly translucent and garlic and onions are soft, 7 – 9 minutes. Place in a bowl and let cool.

3

Place cottage cheese, egg whites, hot sauce, parsley, oregano, and garlic powder in a blender; blend until smooth. Pour into the bowl of cauliflower mixture; mix completely. Spoon mixture evenly into the greased muffin cups and press down so pancakes are even and flat.

4

Bake in the preheated oven until edges and tops are golden and crispy, about 30 minutes.

Nutrition

41 calories
protein 3.3g
carbohydrates 1.8g
fat 2.4g
cholesterol 2.8mg
sodium 120.6mg.

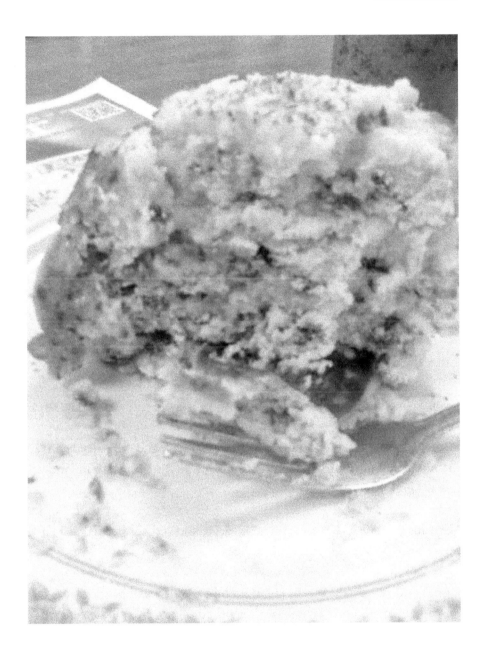

Spinach and Sausage Stuffed Crescents
Prep:20 mins
Cook:30 mins
Additional:10 mins
Servings:8

Ingredients

1 pound spicy bulk pork sausage

¾ (16 ounce) package frozen chopped spinach, thawed and drained

¼ teaspoon red pepper flakes, or more to taste

1 (8 ounce) can refrigerated crescent rolls

1 clove garlic, minced, or more to taste

1 (8 ounce) package reduced-fat cream cheese (Neufchatel), softened

Directions

Preheat oven to 375 degrees F .

2

Heat a large skillet over medium-high heat. Cook and stir sausage in the hot skillet until browned and crumbly, 6 to 8 minutes; drain and discard grease.

3

Mix sausage, cream cheese, spinach, garlic, and red pepper flakes in a bowl.

4

Unroll and separate crescent roll dough into individual portions. Spread equal amounts of the sausage mixture into the middle of each dough portion. Roll and wrap dough around the filling to look like a baseball rather than a crescent roll; arrange onto a baking sheet.

5

Bake in preheated oven until golden brown, about 25 minutes. Cool 10 minutes before serving.

Nutrition

340 calories; protein 14g; carbohydrates 14.2g; fat 25g; cholesterol 53.8mg; sodium 869.2mg.

Beautiful Smoothie (kiwi, banana, apple smoothie amore)

Prep:10 mins
Servings:2

Ingredients

1 apple, roughly chopped
1 teaspoon maca powder
1 banana, broken into chunks
2 kiwifruit, peeled
¼ cup ice, or as desired
2 teaspoons chia seeds
1 ¼ cups milk

Directions

Blend apple, banana, kiwifruit, milk, ice, chia seeds, and maca powder together in a blender until smooth.

Nutrition

232 calories; protein 7.6g; carbohydrates 44.1g; fat 4.5g; cholesterol 12.2mg; sodium 67.4mg.

Dutch Pancakes

Prep:20 mins

Cook:20 mins

Servings:12

Ingredients

6 eggs

2 teaspoons vanilla extract

1 cup milk

2 tablespoons butter, melted

1 ½ cups white sugar

¾ cup buttermilk

½ cup butter

2 tablespoons light corn syrup

1 cup all-purpose flour

1 teaspoon baking soda

Directions

Preheat oven to 400 degrees F . Grease a 9x13 inch baking pan with the melted butter.

2

Place eggs, milk and flour in a blender and whip until smooth. Pour into prepared pan.

3

Bake in preheated oven for 20 minutes, or until golden.

4

In a small saucepan, combine sugar, buttermilk, butter, corn syrup, baking soda; boil for 7 minutes. Remove from heat and stir in vanilla. Spoon over slices of pancake.

Nutrition

283 calories; protein 5.5g; carbohydrates 37.5g; fat 12.7g; cholesterol 120.7mg; sodium 234.8mg.

Mulligatawny

Prep:20 mins
Cook:1 hr
Servings:6

Ingredients

½ cup chopped onion
¼ cup butter
2 stalks celery, chopped
1 carrot, diced
1 ½ tablespoons all-purpose flour
4 cups chicken broth
½ apple, cored and chopped
¼ cup white rice
1 ½ teaspoons curry powder
1 skinless, boneless chicken breast half - cut into cubes
salt to taste
ground black pepper to taste
½ cup heavy cream, heated
1 pinch dried thyme

Directions

Saute onions, celery, carrot, and butter in a large soup pot. Add flour and curry, and cook 5 more minutes. Add chicken stock, mix well, and bring to a boil. Simmer about 1/2 hour.

2

Add apple, rice, chicken, salt, pepper, and thyme. Simmer 15-20 minutes, or until rice is done.

3

When serving, add hot cream.

Nutrition

223 calories; protein 6.9g; carbohydrates 13.5g; fat 15.8g; cholesterol 62.2mg; sodium 733.9mg.

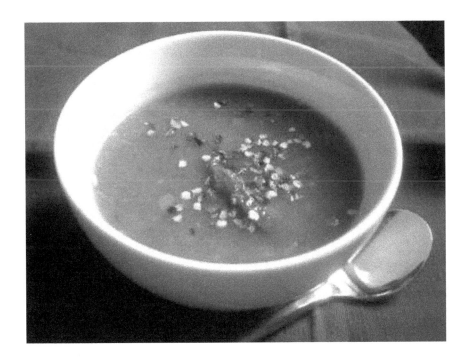

SIMPLE EGGS AND BEANS

YIELD 4 to 6 servings
TIME 30 minutes

Ingredients

2 tablespoons olive oil

Black pepper

½ pound sweet or spicy Italian sausage, casings removed (optional)

4 cups stemmed and packed roughly chopped greens such as spinach, kale or Swiss chard

1 (15-ounce) can chickpeas or white beans, drained and rinsed

2 garlic cloves, finely chopped

Kosher salt

1 (28-ounce) can whole tomatoes, gently crushed by hand

6 large eggs

2 tablespoons mixed herbs, such as Italian parsley and basil, for garnish

1 medium yellow onion, thinly sliced

Grated cheese, such as pecorino or Parmesan, for serving (optional)

Directions

Heat the oven to 375 degrees. Heat the olive oil in a 12-inch ovenproof skillet over medium heat. If using the sausage, add to the pan and cook, breaking it into 1/2-inch pieces, by pressing with the back of spatula or wooden spoon until crisp and cooked through, about 8 minutes. Remove with a slotted spoon and set aside.

Add the onion to the skillet and cook until softened, about 3 to 5 minutes. Add the chickpeas and the garlic and cook until the garlic is fragrant, about 1 minute. Season with salt. Add the sausage back to the pan along with the tomatoes and stir to combine. Bring to a simmer and gradually add in the chopped greens by the handful, tossing together until wilted. Season with salt.

Using a spoon, create hollows in the sauce and gently crack the eggs into each, and season the eggs with salt and pepper. Transfer to the oven and cook until the eggs are set, about 7 to 9 minutes. Scatter the herbs on top along with a tablespoon or two of grated cheese, if using.

Eggs Creamy Melt

Ingredients

1/2 tablespoon butter

1/8 teaspoon kosher salt, or more to taste

4 large eggs

Directions

Melt the butter in a medium non-stick pan over medium-low heat. Crack eggs into a bowl, add a pinch of salt and whisk until well blended.

When the butter begins to bubble, pour in the eggs and immediately use a silicone spatula to swirl in small circles around the pan, without stopping, until the eggs look slightly thickened and very small curds begin to form, about 30 seconds.

Change from making circles to making long sweeps across the pan until you see larger, creamy curds; about 30 seconds.

When the eggs are softly set and slightly runny in places, remove the pan from the heat and leave for a few seconds to finish cooking. Give a final stir and serve immediately. Serve with an extra sprinkle of salt, a grind of black pepper and a few fresh chopped herbs.

Nutrition

Calories 168 / Protein 13 g / Carbohydrate 1 g / Dietary Fiber 0 g / Total Sugars 0 g / Total Fat 12 g / Saturated Fat 5 g / Cholesterol 380 mg

GOAT CHEESE FILING OMELET

Yield:2 servings (serving size: 1 omelet and 1/2 cup vegetables)

Ingredients

4 large eggs
1 tablespoon water
⅛ teaspoon salt
1 teaspoon chopped fresh parsley
½ teaspoon chopped fresh tarragon
¼ teaspoon freshly ground black pepper, divided
¼ cup (1 ounce) crumbled goat cheese
2 teaspoons olive oil, divided
½ cup thinly sliced zucchini
Dash of salt
1 teaspoon chopped fresh chives
½ cup (3 x 1/4–inch) julienne-cut red bell pepper

Directions

Combine eggs and 1 tablespoon water in a bowl, stirring with a whisk. Stir in 1/8 teaspoon pepper and 1/8 teaspoon salt. Combine parsley, tarragon, and goat cheese in a small bowl.

2

Heat 1 teaspoon olive oil in an 8-inch nonstick skillet over medium heat. Add remaining 1/8 teaspoon pepper, zucchini, bell pepper, and dash of salt to pan; cook for 4 minutes or until tender. Remove zucchini mixture from pan; cover and keep warm.

3

Place 1/2 teaspoon oil in skillet. Pour half of the egg mixture into pan, and let egg mixture set slightly (do not stir). Carefully loosen set edges of omelet with a spatula, tipping the pan to pour uncooked egg to the sides. Continue this procedure for about 3 seconds or until almost no runny egg remains. Sprinkle half of cheese mixture evenly over omelet; cook omelet 1 minute or until set. Slide omelet onto plate, folding into thirds. Repeat procedure with remaining 1/2 teaspoon oil, egg mixture, and goat cheese mixture. Sprinkle chives over omelets. Serve with zucchini mixture.

Nutrion

233 calories; fat 17.6g; saturated fat 5.8g; mono fat 7.8g; poly fat 2g; protein 16g; carbohydrates 3.6g; fiber 1g; cholesterol 430mg; iron 2.5mg; sodium 416mg; calcium 84mg.

Berry and Chia Yogurt

Ingredients
1 cup plain nonfat Greek yogurt

1 teaspoon honey

1 Tbsp chia seeds

1 cup fresh or frozen berries

Directions
Combine yogurt and chia seeds in a to-go container.

Mix well.

Add fresh or frozen berries on top of yogurt mixture and lightly drizzle with honey.

Let it sit overnight to allow the flavors to meld and the chia seeds to create a thicker texture.

Nutrition
Calories 300kcal

Total fat 3g

Cholesterol 85 mg

Sodium 85mg

ZUCCHINI PATE

READY IN: 1hr 30mins
SERVES: 4-6

Ingredients

8 ounces zucchini
1 teaspoon white wine vinegar
1 teaspoon salt
1 teaspoon sugar
2 tablespoons chopped parsley
2 tablespoons chopped chives
3 -4 ounces cream cheese
salt and pepper

Directions

Coarsely grate the zucchini, mix with the vinegar, salt and sugar.
Leave this in a sieve, you can line it with cheese cloth if you have it,
cover and leave for an hour or so.
In your food-processor, process the parsley and chives until finely
chopped.
Squeeze the zucchini to get as much moisture out as possible, with just
your hands or whilst in the cheese cloth.
Add the drained zucchini to the food-processor, process until smooth.
Then add the cream cheese, some salt and pepper to taste, process
until it is well combined.
Put the pate in a small bowl, cover and put in the fridge for a few
hours or overnight.
If you line the bowl with cling film you can turn it out of the bowl,
peeling of the cling film, dust the pate with some paprika, then garnish
with some thin cucumber slices around it, but this is optional.
Serve with pita toasts.

Nutrition

Calories: 88.5

Calories from Fat 67 g77 %

Total Fat 7.5 g11 %

Saturated Fat 4.7 g23 %

Cholesterol 23.4 mg7 %

Sodium 651.1 mg27 %

Total Carbohydrate 3.7 g1 %

Dietary Fiber 0.7 g2 %

Sugars 2.1 g8 %

Protein 2.4 g4 %

Pork with Arugula

Total:30 mins
Yield:4

Ingredients

2 tablespoons olive oil
1 1/2 pounds pork tenderloin, cut into 1-inch-thick medallions
Salt and freshly ground pepper
2 tablespoons balsamic vinegar
2 large garlic cloves, minced
1 pound arugula, stems discarded and leaves chopped
1 pound plum tomatoes, chopped
5 ounces thinly sliced prosciutto, finely chopped

Directions

In a very large skillet, heat the olive oil. Add the prosciutto and garlic and cook over moderate heat, stirring, until the garlic is golden, about 4 minutes. Transfer to a plate.

   2

Season the pork medallions with salt and pepper, add them to the skillet and cook over moderately high heat until well browned on the outside and medium within, 4 minutes per side. Transfer the medallions to a plate and keep warm.

   3

Add the balsamic vinegar to the skillet and cook until nearly evaporated, scraping up any browned bits from the bottom of the skillet. Add the arugula and toss until wilted, 2 minutes. Add the tomatoes and the prosciutto and garlic. Cook over high heat for 2 minutes, stirring occasionally; season with salt and pepper. Transfer the arugula to a platter, top with the pork and serve.

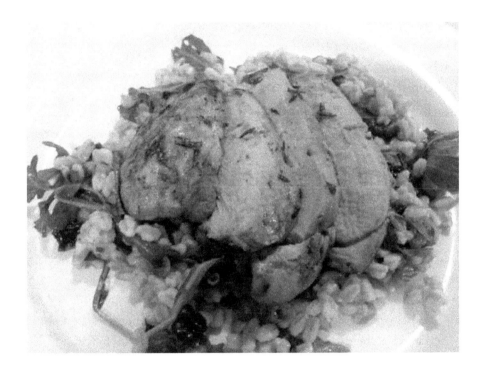

SALMON OMELET

Prep/Total Time: 25 min.
Makes 3 servings

Ingredients

6 eggs
1 salmon fillet (1 inch thick, about 10 ounces)
1/4 teaspoon pepper
1/4 cup finely chopped onion
2 tablespoons butter, divided
1/4 cup finely chopped green pepper
eggs1/4 cup shredded cheddar cheese

Directions

Remove the skin and bones from the salmon; cut into 1/2-in. chunks. In a 10-in. skillet, saute the salmon, onion and green pepper in 1 tablespoon butter. Remove and set aside.

In a small bowl, beat eggs. Melt remaining butter in same skillet over medium heat; add eggs. As eggs set, lift edges, letting uncooked portion flow underneath.

When the eggs are set, spoon salmon mixture over one side, then sprinkle with cheese and pepper; fold omelet over filling. Cover and let stand for 1-1/2 minutes or until the cheese is melted.

If desired, make a tomato rose. With a small sharp knife, peel the skin in a thin continuous strip, starting from the base of the tomato. Roll up tightly, skin side out, from the stem end. Tuck end of strip under rose and place on omelet. From green pepper, cut two leaves. Arrange on each side of tomato rose.

Baked Orange Pecan French Toast

Prep:20 mins

Cook:35 mins

Additional:1 hr

Servings:12

Ingredients

1 cup packed brown sugar

⅓ cup butter, melted

⅓ cup chopped pecans

1 tablespoon confectioners' sugar for dusting

12 (3/4 inch thick) slices French bread

1 teaspoon grated orange zest

1 cup fresh orange juice

2 tablespoons light corn syrup

½ cup 2% milk

3 tablespoons white sugar

1 teaspoon vanilla extract

3 egg whites

2 eggs

1 tablespoon confectioners' sugar for dusting

1 teaspoon ground cinnamon

Directions

In a small bowl, stir together the brown sugar, melted butter, and corn syrup. Pour into a greased 9x13 inch baking dish, and spread evenly. Sprinkle pecans over the sugar mixture. Arrange the bread slices in the bottom of the dish so they are in a snug single layer.

2

In a medium bowl, whisk together the orange zest, orange juice, milk, sugar, cinnamon, vanilla, egg whites, and eggs. Pour this mixture over the bread, pressing on the bread slices to help absorb the liquid. Cover and refrigerate for at least one hour, or overnight.

3

Preheat the oven to 350 degrees F. Remove the cover from the baking dish, and let stand for 20 minutes at room temperature.

4

Bake for 35 minutes in the preheated oven, until golden brown. Dust with confectioners' sugar before serving.

Nutrition

:

235 calories; protein 4.5g; carbohydrates 35.8g; fat 8.8g; cholesterol 45.4mg; sodium 165.8mg.

Derby Pie

Prep:

15 mins

Cook:

44 mins

Additional:

30 mins

Total:

1 hr 29 mins

Servings:

8

Yield:

1 9-inch pie

Ingredients

1 (9 inch) store-bought pie crust, unbaked

3 tablespoons bourbon whiskey

¾ teaspoon instant coffee granules

¾ cup chopped pecans

¾ cup white sugar

3 eggs

¾ cup white corn syrup

6 tablespoons butter, melted

1 ½ teaspoons vanilla extract

¾ cup semisweet chocolate chips

Directions

1

Preheat oven to 425 degrees F (220 degrees C).

2

Press pie crust into a 9-inch pie plate. Prick the bottom of the crust with a fork.

3

Bake pie crust in the preheated oven until it looks dry, 4 to 5 minutes. Let cool. Reduce oven temperature to 350 degrees F (175 degrees C).

4

Pour bourbon whiskey into a small pot; heat over very low heat. Stir in instant coffee until dissolved. Stir in pecans.

5

Beat sugar and eggs together in a bowl until well blended. Beat in corn syrup, melted butter, and vanilla extract. Fold in pecan mixture and chocolate chips. Pour mixture into the pie crust.

6

Bake in the preheated oven until filling is firm and golden brown and crust is lightly browned, 40 to 45 minutes. Cool completely before slicing, at least 30 minutes.

Nutritions
Per Serving: 539 calories; protein 5.4g; carbohydrates 64.3g; fat 30.1g; cholesterol 92.6mg; sodium 225.4mg.

Berry Chia with Yogurt

Prep:

10 mins

Additional:

1 hr 15 mins

Total:

1 hr 25 mins

Servings:

4

Yield:

4 servings

Ingredients

1 cup unsweetened soy milk

1 cup Greek yogurt

2 tablespoons hulled hemp seeds

2 tablespoons ground flax seeds

1 tablespoon honey, or more to taste (Optional)

1 teaspoon ground cinnamon

1 teaspoon vanilla extract

⅔ cup chia seeds

Directions

1

Whisk soy milk and Greek yogurt together in a large sealable container. Stir hemp seeds, flax seeds, honey, cinnamon, and vanilla extract into yogurt mixture.

2

Stir chia seeds into yogurt mixture until seeds are evenly distributed. Cover the container and refrigerate for 15 minutes. Stir mixture until chia seeds are evenly distributed again. Refrigerate until chilled and set, at least 1 hour.

Nutritions

Per Serving: 263 calories; protein 10.4g; carbohydrates 21.1g; fat 15.9g; cholesterol 11.3mg; sodium 68.7mg.

Quinoa Bake with Banana

Prep:

5 mins

Cook:

25 mins

Additional:

30 mins

Total:

1 hr

Servings:

6

Yield:

6 servings

Ingredients

¾ cup quinoa

1 ½ cups water

2 ripe bananas

1 cup whole milk

1 cup coconut milk

4 tablespoons honey, divided

1 tablespoon butter

1 teaspoon ground cinnamon, divided

¼ teaspoon salt

Directions

   1

Rinse quinoa in a paper towel-lined colander until water is no longer milky. Transfer quinoa to a saucepan, add 1 1/2 cups water and soak for 30 minutes.

2

Bring quinoa and water to a boil, reduce heat to low, cover, and simmer until water is absorbed, about 15 minutes.

3

Blend bananas, whole milk, coconut milk, 3 tablespoons honey, butter, 1/2 teaspoon cinnamon, and salt together in a blender until smooth.

4

Stir milk mixture into quinoa, raise heat to medium; cook and stir constantly until pudding becomes thick, about 10 minutes.

5

Transfer pudding to serving dish and refrigerate until cold, about 1 hour. Drizzle 1 tablespoon honey over pudding; sprinkle with 1/2 teaspoon cinnamon.

Nutritions
Per Serving: 278 calories; protein 5.6g; carbohydrates 38.7g; fat 12.7g; cholesterol 9.2mg; sodium 135.6mg.

Pine Nut Macaroons

Servings:

60

Yield:

5 dozen

Ingredients

1 pound almond paste
1 ¼ cups white sugar
4 egg whites
4 cups pine nuts

Directions

1

Preheat oven to 350 degrees F (175 degrees C). Grease cookie sheets.

2

Break almond paste into pieces and mix together with sugar, using your hands to crumble paste. In a separate bowl, separate the eggs and beat the whites into soft peaks. Slowly add to almond paste mixture and mix until just blended.

3

Place pine nuts into bowl. Roll dough into 1-inch balls and press into nuts. Coat evenly and place on cookie sheets about 1 inch apart.

4

Bake 15 to 17 minutes, until lightly golden. Let cool on cookie sheets for 5 minutes, then transfer to racks.

Nutritions

Per Serving: 103 calories; protein 3.1g; carbohydrates 9.1g; fat 6.7g; sodium 4.7mg.

Egg in a Pepper

Prep:

5 mins

Cook:

5 mins

Total:

10 mins

Servings:

1

Yield:

1 serving

Ingredients

1 large egg
1 (1/4 inch thick) ring bell pepper
salt and ground black pepper to taste

Directions

1

Heat a non-stick skillet over medium heat. Place bell pepper ring in the hot skillet. Crack egg into bell pepper ring; cook until bottom holds together and corners are browned, 2 to 3 minutes. Flip and cook until desired doneness is reached, 2 to 3 minutes more; season with salt and ground black pepper.

Nutritions

Per Serving: 74 calories; protein 6.4g; carbohydrates 0.8g; fat 5g; cholesterol 186mg; sodium 225.3mg.

Toast and Tuna

Prep:

5 mins

Cook:

25 mins

Total:

30 mins

Servings:

3

Yield:

3 servings

Ingredients

1 (10.75 ounce) can condensed cream of mushroom soup

2 hard-cooked eggs, sliced

1 (5 ounce) can tuna, drained

6 slices whole wheat bread

Directions

1

Make cream of mushroom soup according to the directions on the can.

2

Stir in canned tuna and egg slices. Heat thoroughly. Meanwhile, toast bread slices.

3

Spoon tuna mixture over slices of whole wheat toast. Serve.

Nutritions

Per Serving: 317 calories; protein 20.9g; carbohydrates 32g; fat 11.8g; cholesterol 153.9mg; sodium 987.1mg.

Greek Yogurt

Prep:
10 mins
Additional:
6 mins
Total:
16 mins
Servings:
6
Yield:
6 servings

Ingredients

coffee filters, or as needed
1 (32 ounce) container plain yogurt

Directions
1
Line a colander with coffee filters and set it in a large bowl. Add yogurt and cover with a clean kitchen towel. Place in the refrigerator for 6 hours to overnight; the fluid from the yogurt will collect in the bottom of the bowl.

2
Scoop yogurt out of the coffee filters and back into the original container for storage. Discard accumulated fluid or reserve for other use.

Nutritions

Per Serving: 95 calories; protein 7.9g; carbohydrates 10.7g; fat 2.3g; cholesterol 9.1mg; sodium 105.9mg.

CHAPTER 4: LUNCH

ITALIAN prosciutto wraps mozzarella balls

INGREDIENTS

Marinara Sauce 750g
Baguette 750 1 sliced
¼ Butter, softened
2 minced/ grated Cloves garlic
1 Pound Mozzarella Balls
1 Tablespoon Olive Oil
¼ cup grated (optional)
6 ounces, cut in half Prosciutto

Directions:

Spread the mixture of the butter and garlic over the baguette slices and toast until lightly golden brown.

Meanwhile, wrap the mozzarella in prosciutto.

Heat the oil in a pan over medium-high heat, add the prosciutto wrapped mozzarella and cook until lightly golden brown, about a minute per side, and set aside.

Add Pomì Marinara Sauce and parmesan to the pan and heat until the cheese has melted in.

Add the prosciutto wrapped mozzarella and transfer to a preheated 425F oven to bake until the sauce is bubbling and the mozzarella has melted, about 5-10 minutes, before removing from the oven, sprinkling on the basil and enjoying with the garlic crostini.

Caramelized Onions

Prep:10 mins
Cook:25 mins
Servings:4

Ingredients

6 slices bacon, chopped
2 tablespoons molasses
¼ teaspoon salt
¼ teaspoon pepper
2 sweet onions, cut into thin strips

Directions

Place bacon in a heavy skillet. Cook over medium-high heat until crisp.
Remove bacon, reserving 1 tablespoon drippings in skillet. Crumble
bacon, and set aside.
Cook onions in reserved drippings for 15 minutes, or until onion is
soft and caramel colored. Stir in molasses, salt and pepper. Place in a
serving dish, and sprinkle with crumbled bacon.

Nutrition

244 calories; protein 5.5g; carbohydrates 13g; fat 19g; cholesterol
28.6mg; sodium 501.2mg.

ITALIAN MEATBALLS

Prep:20 mins
Cook:35 mins
Additional:1 hr 20 mins
Servings:30

Ingredients

⅓ cup plain bread crumbs
2 tablespoons olive oil
1 onion, diced
½ cup milk
1 pound ground beef
1 pound ground pork
¼ bunch fresh parsley, chopped
3 cloves garlic, crushed
2 teaspoons salt
2 eggs
1 teaspoon ground black pepper
1 teaspoon dried Italian herb seasoning
½ teaspoon red pepper flakes
2 tablespoons grated Parmesan cheese

Directions

Cover a baking sheet with foil and spray lightly with cooking spray.
Soak bread crumbs in milk in a small bowl for 20 minutes.
Heat olive oil in a skillet over medium heat. Cook and stir onions in
hot oil until translucent, about 20 minutes.
Mix beef and pork together in a large bowl. Stir onions, bread crumb
mixture, eggs, parsley, garlic, salt, black pepper, red pepper flakes,
Italian herb seasoning, and Parmesan cheese into meat mixture with a

rubber spatula until combined. Cover and refrigerate for about one hour.

Preheat an oven to 425 degrees F.

Using wet hands, form meat mixture into balls about 1 1/2 inches in diameter. Arrange onto prepared baking sheet.

Bake in the preheated oven until browned and cooked through, 15 to 20 minutes.

Nutrition

82 calories; protein 6.2g; carbohydrates 1.7g; fat 5.5g; cholesterol 32.3mg; sodium 192.1mg.

Cabbage Onion Quiche

Cook: 1 hour 15 minutes, including baking

INGREDIENTS

2 tablespoons extra-virgin olive oil

½ medium cabbage (1 pound), cored and shredded (about 5 cups shredded cabbage)

 Salt to taste

½ teaspoon caraway seeds

1 cup chopped spring onion

2 whole eggs

1 (9-inch) whole wheat pâte brisée pie crust fully baked and cooled

½ teaspoon salt

 Freshly ground pepper

2 egg yolks

⅔ cup milk

3 ounces Gruyère, grated, or 1 ounce Parmesan and 2 ounces Gruyère, grated (3/4 cup grated cheese)

Directions

Preheat oven to 350 degrees.

Heat olive oil over medium heat in a large, heavy skillet and add onions. Cook, stirring often, until tender, about 5 minutes. Add a generous pinch of salt and continue to cook 5 minutes, until beginning to color. Add cabbage and cook, stirring often, until cabbage wilts, about 5 minutes. Add another pinch of salt and caraway seeds and continue to cook for another 7-8 minutes, until cabbage is sweet, cooked down, lightly colored and very tender. Taste, adjust salt, and add freshly ground pepper. Remove from heat.

Beat together egg yolks and eggs in a medium bowl. Set tart pan on a baking sheet to allow for easy handling. Using a pastry brush, lightly brush the bottom of the crust with some of the beaten egg and place in the oven for 5 minutes. (The egg seals the crust so that it won't become soggy when it comes into contact with the custard.)

Add salt (I use 1/2 teaspoon), pepper, and milk to remaining eggs and whisk together.

Spread cabbage and onion in an even layer in the crust. Sprinkle cheese evenly on top. Very slowly pour in the egg custard over the filling. If your tart pan has low edges, you may not need all of it to fill the quiche, and you want to keep the custard from spilling over. Place quiche, on baking sheet, in oven and bake for 30 to 35 minutes, until set and just beginning to color on top. Remove from oven and allow to sit for at least 10 minutes before serving.

Pasta with Cauliflowers

Prep:20 mins
Cook:30 mins
Servings:8

Ingredients

1 medium head cauliflower, cut into bite-sized florets
2 tablespoons olive oil, or more to taste
¼ teaspoon salt
¼ teaspoon ground black pepper
1 (16 ounce) package penne pasta
5 cloves garlic, peeled and smashed
¼ cup lemon juice
¼ cup seasoned bread crumbs
1 teaspoon ground cayenne pepper
2 tablespoons salted butter
1 cup grated Parmesan cheese

Directions

Preheat the oven to 425 degrees F .
Toss cauliflower with garlic cloves, olive oil, salt, and pepper in a large bowl. Spread out in an even layer on a baking sheet.
Roast in the preheated oven, tossing at least twice, until cauliflower is tender, about 30 minutes.
Meanwhile, bring a large pot of lightly salted water to a boil. Add penne and cook, stirring occasionally, until tender yet firm to the bite, about 11 minutes.
Mix Parmesan cheese, bread crumbs, and cayenne pepper together in a bowl; set aside.

Drain pasta, reserving 1/2 cup cooking water. Transfer pasta to a serving bowl and add cauliflower and butter. Stir in cooking water, a little at a time, until desired creaminess is reached. Add lemon juice and bread crumb mixture, toss, and serve.

Nutrition

333 calories; protein 13.2g; carbohydrates 48.2g; fat 10.7g; cholesterol 16.5mg; sodium 332.4mg.

Mujadara (Lentils and Rice with Caramelized Onions)

Prep Time: 25 minutes
Cook Time: 35 minutes
Servings: 4

INGREDIENTS

4 medium cloves garlic, smashed and peeled
2 bay leaves
1 tablespoon ground cumin
1 ¾ teaspoons fine sea salt, divided
5 cups water
1 cup regular brown or green lentils**, picked over for debris, rinsed and drained
⅓ cup extra-virgin olive oil
Freshly ground black pepper
2 medium-to-large yellow onions, halved and thinly sliced
½ cup thinly sliced green onions (from 1 bunch), divided
½ cup chopped fresh cilantro or flat-leaf parsley, divided
1 cup brown* basmati rice (regular, not quick-cooking), rinsed and drained
Plain whole-milk or Greek yogurt, for serving
Spicy sauce, for serving

Directions

In a large Dutch oven or soup pot, combine the garlic, bay leaves, cumin, 1 ½ teaspoons of the salt and about 20 twists of freshly ground black pepper. Add the water and bring the mixture to a boil over medium-high heat.

Once boiling, stir in the rice and reduce the heat to medium. Cover and cook, stirring occasionally and adjusting the heat as necessary to maintain a controlled simmer, for 10 minutes.

Stir in the lentils and let the mixture return to a simmer. Cover again, reduce the heat to medium-low, and cook until the liquid is absorbed and the rice and lentils are tender, about 20 to 23 minutes.

Meanwhile, warm the olive oil in a large (12-inch) skillet over medium-high heat. When it's warm enough that a slice of onion sizzles on contact, add the remaining onions. Stir to combine.

Stir only every 3-4 minutes or so at first, then more often once the onions at the edges of the pan start browning. If the onions are browning before they have softened, dial down the heat to give them more time. Cook until the onions are deeply caramelized and starting to crisp at the edges, about 20 to 30 minutes. In the meantime, line a large plate or cutting board with a couple paper towels.

Using a slotted spoon or fish spatula, transfer the onions to the lined plate and spread them evenly across. Sprinkle the remaining ¼ teaspoon salt over the onions. They'll crisp up as they cool.

When the lentils and rice are done cooking, drain off any excess water (if there is any) and return the mixture to the pot, off the heat. Lay a kitchen towel across the top of the pot to absorb steam, then cover the pot and let it rest for 10 minutes.

Remove the lid, discard the bay leaves, and smash the garlic cloves against the side of the pan with a fork. Add about ¾ths of the green onions and cilantro, reserving the rest for garnish. Gently stir and fluff the rice with a fork. Season to taste with additional salt and pepper, if necessary.

Transfer the rice and lentil mixture to a large serving platter or bowl. Top with the caramelized onions and the remaining green onions and cilantro. Serve hot, warm or at room temperature, with yogurt and spicy sauce (optional) on the side.

Macaroni & Cheese

Prep:10 mins
Cook:12 mins
Servings:4

Ingredients

1 (6 ounce) box Macaroni & Mild Cheddar Cheese
½ cup shredded sharp Cheddar cheese
2 ounces Organic Milk
1 cup Cooked broccoli florets
1 tablespoon butter

Directions

Cook the noodles according to the package directions.
Drain and pour into a large bowl.
Immediately add the butter and shredded cheese. Stir to mix while still hot. The cheese should melt. If it doesn't, put the mixture back in the pan and heat for another minute on medium, stirring constantly until the cheese has melted.
Add the cheese mix, milk, and broccoli, if using. Stir until combined.

Nutrition

255 calories; protein 10.1g; carbohydrates 33g; fat 9.3g; cholesterol 24.6mg; sodium 482.2mg.

Mahi Mahi Ceviche

Prep:30 mins
Additional:1 hr
Servings:6

Ingredients

¾ pound mahi mahi fillets, diced, or more to taste
⅓ cup lime juice
1 tablespoon minced jalapeno pepper
½ teaspoon salt
⅓ cup lemon juice
1 pinch cayenne pepper
½ cup diced avocados
½ cup peeled and seeded diced cucumber
1 pinch dried oregano
½ cup diced orange segments
2 tablespoons radishes, sliced
1 tablespoon chopped cilantro
1 tablespoon olive oil
½ cup chopped fresh chives

Directions

Stir mahi mahi, lime juice, lemon juice, jalapeno pepper, salt, oregano, and cayenne pepper together in a bowl. Press down fish to completely immerse in liquid. Cover the bowl with plastic wrap and press plastic wrap down so that it is touching the fish. Refrigerate for at least 1 hour, or up to 6 hours.

Stir avocado, cucumber, orange, chives, radish, cilantro, and olive oil into mahi mahi mixture until completely coated. Season with salt.

Nutrition

117 calories; protein 11.4g; carbohydrates 6.5g; fat 5.6g; cholesterol 41.5mg; sodium 247mg.

Snickers Caramel Apple Salad

Prep:10 mins
Additional:30 mins
Servings:12

Ingredients

1 (8 ounce) container frozen whipped topping, thawed
1 (8 ounce) can crushed pineapple
1 (3.4 ounce) package instant butterscotch pudding mix
1 cup skinless peanuts
2 cups chopped apples

Directions

Stir whipped topping, pineapple, and butterscotch pudding mix
together in a bowl until smooth. Fold apples and peanuts into pudding
mixture until salad is well mixed.
Refrigerate salad until completely chilled, at least 30 minutes.

Nutrition

181 calories; protein 3.2g; carbohydrates 20g; fat 10.8g; sodium
227.7mg.

Crispy Chicken Cutlets

Prep:25 mins
Cook:20 mins
Additional:30 mins
Servings:2

Ingredients

2 skinless, boneless chicken breast halves
¼ teaspoon salt
2 tablespoons cornstarch
1 teaspoon salt
½ teaspoon freshly ground black pepper
3 tablespoons all-purpose flour
1 pinch white sugar
¼ cup medium sherry
1 cup chicken broth
2 tablespoons butter
1 Granny Smith apple - cored, peeled, and cut into 1/2-inch thick wedges
1 tablespoon butter
⅓ cup light brown sugar
⅓ cup light brown sugar
1 dash Marsala wine

Directions

Sprinkle chicken breasts with 1/4 teaspoon salt, or as needed, on both sides. Place onto a rack, cover, and refrigerate for 30 minutes. Remove from refrigerator, and cut in half lengthwise on a slight diagonal to make 4 equal-size pieces. Place the chicken pieces between two sheets of heavy plastic (resealable freezer bags work well) on a solid, level surface. Firmly pound the chicken with the smooth side of a meat mallet to make 4 cutlets about 1/4 inch thick.

Preheat oven to 200 degrees F .

Mix together flour, cornstarch, 1 teaspoon of salt, black pepper, and sugar in a shallow bowl. Place each cutlet into the flour mixture to coat; shake off excess flour. Melt 2 tablespoons of butter in a skillet over medium heat until foam disappears, and gently lay the coated cutlets into the butter. Cook until golden brown on both sides, about 3 minutes per side. Remove the chicken, and set aside on an oven-proof plate in the preheated oven to stay warm.

Pour the sherry into the skillet and bring to a boil, scraping and dissolving all the brown flavor bits from the bottom of the skillet. Cook until the sherry is reduced to half its volume, about 5 minutes, and stir in the chicken broth; add the apple slices to the skillet. Cook, stirring occasionally, until the apples are soft and the sherry mixture is reduced by half. Stir in the brown sugar, 1 tablespoon of butter, and the Marsala wine until the sugar is dissolved and the sauce is thick. Return the chicken cutlets to the sauce, together with any juice from the plate, and turn to cover cutlets with sauce. Simmer about 2 minutes per side, and serve 2 cutlets per serving, topped with apple slices and sauce.

Nutrition

586 calories; protein 21.3g; carbohydrates 61.2g; fat 27.8g; cholesterol 112.9mg; sodium 1981.5mg.

Cod Balls

Cook: 20 mins
Prep: 5 mins
Servings: 4

Ingredients

2 eggs, lightly beaten
2 lbs. of cod filet
1/2 cup minced fresh parsley
1/2 cup of minced onion
A dusting of flour to roll balls in
Oil for deep frying (A mix of olive oil and canola works well, although the traditional recipes call for corn oil)

Directions

Steam the cod until it is cooked through and flaky. The easiest way is to put pieces of the cod of it into a steamer basket over a pot of boiling water. When it is fully cooked, remove the cod from the steamer, put it in a large bowl, and flake the meat. Put the flaked cod in the refrigerator to chill.

When the fish has cooled, add the potatoes, parsley, minced onions, and eggs to the bowl and mix thoroughly. If you are not going to roll the balls right away, put the mixture in the refrigerator until you are ready. The mixture forms better balls when it is cold.

With your hands, roll the mixture into approximately 2-inch balls. Put some flour onto a plate. Lightly roll each ball into the flour.

Heat the oil (about 2 inches high) in a heavy pot. When it is hot, put a few of the balls into the oil. (To check the oil temperature, drop a tiny bit of mixture into the pot. If it sizzles and fries, it's ready.) You will need to do this in batches because overcrowding will make it hard to turn the balls.

Roll the balls around with a spoon to ensure that they brown on all sides. When they are golden brown, remove them from the oil with a slotted spoon.

Put the balls on paper towels to drain and serve immediately.

Basil Vea Rolls

Prep 20 min
Cook 30 min
Serves 6

Ingredients

Fresh basil
1 cup(s)
Garlic
1 clove(s), chopped
Pine nuts
2 tbs
Grated parmesan cheese
2 tbs
Olive oil
1 tbs
Lemon juice
1 tbs
Reduced-fat ricotta cheese
180 g
Lean veal leg steak
600 g, fat trimmed, (buy750g)
Red onion
1 medium, finely chopped
Garlic
2 clove(s), crushed
Tomato passata
2 cup(s), (500ml)
Fresh basil
2 tbs, shredded
Oil spray
1 x 3 second spray(s)

Directions

Preheat oven to 180°C or 160°C fan-forced. Place basil leaves, garlic, nuts and parmesan in a food processor and process until chopped finely. Add oil, juice and 1 tablespoon water, processing until almost smooth. Combine pesto and ricotta in a bowl. Season with salt and black pepper.

Pound each steak to 3mm thick with a meat mallet between 2 pieces of baking paper. Cut each steak in half lengthwise to make 12 and place on a flat surface. Divide pesto ricotta evenly among steaks, spreading to cover. Tightly roll steaks from short end to enclose filling. Secure with a toothpick.

Lightly spray a large non-stick frying pan with oil and heat over high heat. Cook veal for 2 minutes each side or until lightly browned. Arrange veal in 2L (8-cup) capacity ovenproof dish.

Lightly spray same frying pan with oil and heat over medium heat. Add red onion and cook, stirring, for 3–5 minutes or until softened. Add garlic and cook, stirring, for 1 minute or until fragrant. Add passata and bring to the boil. Reduce heat to low and simmer for 5 minutes or until sauce thickens slightly. Stir in shredded basil. Pour sauce over veal. Cover with foil and bake for 10–12 minutes or until cooked to your liking. Remove toothpicks and serve veal rolls drizzled with sauce.

Zucchini Sautè

Prep:15 mins
Cook:15 mins
Servings:6

Ingredients

1 tablespoon olive oil
½ red onion, diced
salt and pepper to taste
½ pound fresh mushrooms, sliced
1 teaspoon Italian seasoning
1 tomato, diced
1 clove garlic, minced
4 zucchini, halved and sliced

Directions

Heat oil in a large skillet over medium heat. Saute onion with salt and pepper for 2 minutes. Stir in zucchini and mushrooms. When zucchini begins to soften, add tomatoes, garlic and Italian seasoning. Cook until heated through.

Nutrition

68 calories; protein 2.8g; carbohydrates 9.2g; fat 3.2g; sodium 99.1mg.

Honey Molasses Pork

Serves:6
Prep:2 Hr 10 Min
Cook: 30 Min

Directions

In a bowl combine all ingredients except pork chops, stir well. In a large bowl put the chops and pour marinade over the top, making sure to cover them all. Every 1/2 move them around in the marinade. Marinade 2hr or longer.

Turn grill to medium. Place chops on a grill pan and cook 16-20 minutes or until done. Through out grilling, brush marinade over chops.

Jammin' Jambalaya

Prep:20 mins
Cook:45 mins
Servings:6

Ingredients

2 tablespoons peanut oil, divided
10 ounces andouille sausage, sliced into rounds
1 pound boneless skinless chicken breasts, cut into 1 inch pieces
1 onion, diced
1 tablespoon Cajun seasoning
1 small green bell pepper, diced
3 cloves garlic, minced
1 (16 ounce) can crushed Italian tomatoes
½ teaspoon red pepper flakes
2 stalks celery, diced
½ teaspoon ground black pepper
1 teaspoon salt
2 teaspoons Worcestershire sauce
1 teaspoon file powder
½ teaspoon hot pepper sauce
1 ¼ cups uncooked white rice
2 ½ cups chicken broth

Directions

Heat 1 tablespoon of peanut oil in a large heavy Dutch oven over
medium heat. Season the sausage and chicken pieces with Cajun
seasoning. Saute sausage until browned. Remove with slotted spoon,
and set aside. Add 1 tablespoon peanut oil, and saute chicken pieces

until lightly browned on all sides. Remove with a slotted spoon, and set aside.

In the same pot, saute onion, bell pepper, celery and garlic until tender. Stir in crushed tomatoes, and season with red pepper, black pepper, salt, hot pepper sauce, Worcestershire sauce and file powder. Stir in chicken and sausage. Cook for 10 minutes, stirring occasionally.

Stir in the rice and chicken broth. Bring to a boil, reduce heat, and simmer for 20 minutes, or until liquid is absorbed.

Nutrition

465 calories; protein 28.1g; carbohydrates 42.4g; fat 19.8g; cholesterol 73.1mg; sodium 1632.7mg.

Mince with Basil

0:30 Prep
0:15 Cook
6 Servings

INGREDIENTS

1 iceberg lettuce
2 tablespoons vegetable oil
500g lean beef mince
1 tablespoon white sugar
3 long red chillies, sliced
4 cloves garlic, finely chopped
2 tablespoons fish sauce
1 tablespoon oyster sauce
1/2 cup Massel chicken style liquid stock
1/3 cup basil leaves, shredded
3 green onions, thinly sliced
Select all ingredients

Directions

Remove core from lettuce. Cut in half lengthways and place into a large bowl of cold water. Allow to stand for 30 minutes. This loosens the leaves and enables easy peeling to form cups.
Heat oil in a large frypan over high heat. Add half the mince and cook, stirring continuously, until well-browned. Remove and repeat with remaining mince.
Return mince to pan and add chillies, garlic, fish sauce, sugar, oyster sauce, and stock. Stir until well-combined. Bring to the boil. Reduce the heat to medium-low and simmer. Add green onions and cook for 4 minutes.

Remove from heat and fold through basil. Spoon the chilli mince beef into the lettuce cups and serve immediately.

Chickpea Curry

Prep:15 mins
Cook:35 mins
Servings:4

Ingredients

1 tablespoon butter

3 cloves garlic, minced

3 teaspoons curry powder

2 teaspoons garam masala

1 onion, chopped

½ teaspoon white sugar

½ teaspoon ground ginger

¼ teaspoon ground turmeric

¼ teaspoon salt

¼ teaspoon pepper

¼ cup ground almonds

½ teaspoon ground paprika

1 (15 ounce) can garbanzo beans, drained

1 (14 ounce) can coconut milk

1 tomato, chopped

⅓ cup milk

2 tablespoons ketchup

2 tablespoons sour cream

2 potatoes, chopped

2 cubes chicken bouillon

Directions

Melt the butter over medium heat in a large saucepan. Cook and stir the onion and garlic in the melted butter for about 5 minutes, until onion is translucent. Sprinkle in curry powder, garam masala, paprika, sugar, ginger, turmeric, salt, and pepper. Continue to cook and stir 4 more minutes, until spices are lightly toasted.

Mix in the garbanzo beans, potatoes, coconut milk, tomato, milk, ketchup, sour cream, and bouillon cubes. Simmer the curry over medium-low heat for about 25 minutes, until the potatoes are tender. Stir in ground almonds to thicken.

Nutrition

505 calories; protein 11.9g; carbohydrates 49.7g; fat 31.8g; cholesterol 12.7mg; sodium 1072.6mg.

Cote d'Ivoire Fish

Serves: 4 adults

Ingredients

4 lbs Whole Nile Perch, cleaned and scaled
2 tomatoes, cut into 4 pieces
2 tablespoons oil
2 limes, juice of
2 medium yellow onions, roughly cut
4 cloves garlic, crushed
1 scotch bonnet pepper, stemmed and roughly chopped
1 Jumbo cube, crushed (or shrimp flavored Maggi cube, if Jumbo is unavailable in your area)
salt and freshly ground black pepper to taste
1 bunch flat-leaf parsley, roughly chopped
Garnish
4-6 sprigs fresh flat-leaf parsley
2-3 fresh limes, cut into wedges

Directions

Wash the fish gently with cold water. Drain, and pat dry with paper towels.
Slit the fish (cuts should be about 1/2-inch deep, 3-4 inches in length) 3 times on each side and massage the fish (inside and out) with the fresh lime juice.
Put tomatoes, onions, pepper, garlic, parsley and oil in the bowl of a food processor fitted with the steel chopping blade. Season generously with salt, pepper and the crushed seasoning cube. Process until mixture forms a paste, adding additional oil, as needed.
Massage the fish generously with this mixture, ensuring that you push some into the cuts on both sides of the fish.

Leave the fish to marinate in the refrigerator for 60 minutes.

Remove fish from marinade, reserving marinade juices, and grill over charcoal fire. (Alternately, fish can be broiled in the oven or cooked on a gas grill. However, the charcoal adds an additional layer of authentic flavor to the finished dish.)

Meanwhile, add remaining marinade liquid to a small saucepan and cook over medium heat until mixture reaches a boil. Allow to simmer for 5-7 minutes to ensure marinade is thoroughly cooked.

Serve with sauce, attiéké, and Ivorian salad. Garnish with sprigs of fresh parsley, and lime wedges.

JOLLOF RICE

Prep:20 mins

Cook:1 hr

Servings:8

Ingredients

1 tablespoon olive oil

1 large onion, sliced

½ (6 ounce) can tomato paste

1 teaspoon salt

2 (14.5 ounce) cans stewed tomatoes

¼ teaspoon black pepper

¼ teaspoon cayenne pepper

½ teaspoon red pepper flakes

1 tablespoon Worcestershire sauce

2 cups water

1 (3 pound) whole chicken, cut into 8 pieces

1 teaspoon chopped fresh rosemary

1 cup uncooked white rice

½ pound fresh green beans, trimmed and snapped into 1 to 2 inch pieces

¼ teaspoon ground nutmeg

1 cup diced carrots

Directions

Pour oil into large saucepan. Cook onion in oil over medium-low heat until translucent.

Stir in stewed tomatoes and tomato paste, and season with salt, black pepper, cayenne pepper, red pepper flakes, Worcestershire sauce and rosemary. Cover, and bring to a boil. Reduce heat, stir in water, and add chicken pieces. Simmer for 30 minutes.

Stir in rice, carrots, and green beans, and season with nutmeg. Bring to a boil, then reduce heat to low. Cover, and simmer until the chicken is fork-tender and the rice is cooked, 27 to 30 minutes.

Nutrition

332 calories; protein 19.8g; carbohydrates 33.5g; fat 13.4g; cholesterol 46.1mg; sodium 712.6mg

Frosted Grapes

Prep:5 mins
Additional:1 hr
Servings:8

Ingredients

2 pounds red seedless grapes
1 (3 ounce) package cherry flavored mix

Directions

Pluck grapes from their stems and rinse in a colander. Pour the gelatin mix onto a plate. Place grapes on the plate one handful at a time and roll around until coated. Transfer to a pretty dish and refrigerate for 1 hour to allow the gelatin to set.

Nutrition

119 calories; protein 1.7g; carbohydrates 29.2g; fat 0.7g; sodium 50mg.

Giblet Gravy

Prep:10 mins
Cook:2 hrs 15 mins
Servings:16

Ingredients

1 turkey neck and giblets
2 large white onions, sliced
1 cup sliced carrots
1 cup dry white wine
½ cup celery leaves
6 cloves garlic, peeled
6 cups chicken broth
½ cup turkey drippings
¾ cup all-purpose flour
6 tablespoons butter, softened
1 bay leaf
salt and ground black pepper to taste

Directions

Cut turkey neck in half. Set liver aside.
Combine neck, giblets, broth, onions, carrots, wine, celery, garlic, and bay leaf in a pot. Bring to a boil. Reduce heat and simmer for 1 hour and 30 minutes. Add liver and simmer for 30 minutes more.
Mix flour and butter together to form a thick paste.
Remove and discard neck and giblets. Strain broth, pressing vegetables to extract liquid. Discard vegetables. Add turkey drippings. Add flour mixture gradually and stir until smooth. Bring to a boil and cook until desired thickness is reached, 8 to 10 minutes. Season with salt and pepper.

Nutrition

180 calories; protein 4.7g; carbohydrates 8.4g; fat 12.9g; cholesterol 64.3mg; sodium 496.7mg.

Monk-Fish Curry

SERVES 4
COOKS IN55 MINUTES

Ingredients

500 g monkfish , skinned, deboned (your fishmonger can do this for you)
1 teaspoon ground turmeric
200 g brown rice
1 x 400 ml tin of light coconut milk
2 limes
SAUCE
2 onions
2 cloves of garlic
2 fresh green chillies
10 ripe medium tomatoes, on the vine
groundnut oil
1 small handful of fresh curry leaves
5cm piece of ginger
3 cardamom pods
2 teaspoons brown mustard seeds
1 teaspoon fenugreek seeds
½ teaspoon ground turmeric
1 teaspoon cumin seeds
1 knob of tamarind paste or 1 teaspoon tamarind syrup

Directions

Slice the monkfish into large chunks and pop in a non-reactive bowl, along with the turmeric, lime zest and juice and a large pinch of sea salt.

Mix together to coat the fish, then leave in the fridge for at least 1 hour.

Add the rice to a pan with 100ml of the coconut milk and 300ml of salted water, then cook according to the packet directions.

To make your sauce, peel and finely slice the onions and garlic, peel and finely chop the ginger, then slice the chillies. Roughly chop the tomatoes, keeping them separate.

Heat a large casserole pan over a medium–high heat and add a splash of oil, the onion, ginger, garlic, chillies and curry leaves. Cook for 5 to 10 minutes, or until the onion is softened and coloured.

Smash the cardamom pods in a pestle and mortar, then stir them into the pan along with the mustard seeds, cumin, fenugreek and turmeric. Fry for 1 minute.

Stir in the chopped tomatoes, tamarind paste or syrup, the remaining 300ml of coconut milk and 100ml of water, then simmer for 10 minutes, or until the tomatoes begin to break down and the sauce reduces.

Add the monkfish to the sauce and simmer until the fish is cooked through and opaque. Remove and discard the cardamom pods, then serve with the rice on the side.

Vegetable Masala

Prep:10 mins
Cook:20 mins
Servings:4

Ingredients

2 potatoes, peeled and cubed
10 French-style green beans, chopped
1 quart cold water
½ cup frozen green peas, thawed
1 carrot, chopped
1 teaspoon salt
½ teaspoon ground turmeric
1 tablespoon vegetable oil
1 teaspoon ground cumin
1 onion, finely chopped
2 tomatoes - blanched, peeled and chopped
1 teaspoon mustard seed
1 teaspoon garam masala
½ teaspoon garlic powder
½ teaspoon chili powder
½ teaspoon ground ginger
1 sprig cilantro leaves, for garnish

Directions

Place potatoes, carrots and green beans in the cold water. Allow to soak while you prepare the rest of the vegetables; drain.
In a microwave safe dish place the potatoes, carrots, green beans, peas, salt and turmeric. Cook for 8 minutes.
Heat oil in a large skillet over medium heat. Cook mustard seeds and cumin; when seeds start to sputter and pop, add the onion and saute

until transparent. Stir in the tomatoes, garam masala, ginger, garlic and chili powder; saute 3 minutes. Add the cooked vegetables to the tomato mixture and saute 1 minute. Garnish with cilantro leaves.

Nutrition

168 calories; protein 4.2g; carbohydrates 29.8g; fat 4.3g; sodium 641.3mg.

Jicama Noodles

PREP TIME10 mins
COOK TIME25 mins
SERVINGS: 5

INGREDIENTS

1 large jicama
olive oil to drizzle (about 2 tbsp)
2 teaspoon cayenne pepper
1 tbsp onion powder
2 teaspoon chili powder
salt to tast

DIRECTIONS

Preheat the oven to 405 degrees.
Lay out your jicama noodles and snip them with a scissor to divide
into smaller sized noodles, similar to shoestring fries.
When done, lay your noodles onto two large baking trays, drizzle with
olive oil and toss together to combine and coat noodles.
Season with a generous amount of salt and then evenly season with
onion powder, cayenne pepper and chili powder. Toss again to
combine and then lay them out, trying hard not to crowd them.
Bake in the oven for 15 minutes, turn over and bake another 10-15
minutes or until they reach your doneness preference. Divide onto
plates and enjoy as a snack or a side dish!

GLAZED SALMON

Prep 20 mins
Cook 40 mins
Servings 3

Ingredients

4 salmon fillets
170g of maple syrup
vegetable oil
1 lime, juiced
toasted sesame seeds
15g of soy sauce
VEGETABLES
8 asparagus spears, peeled
8 white asparagus spears, peeled
150g of fresh peas
150g of fresh broad beans, podded
8 wild asparagus spears
baby salad leaves
vegetable oil
coriander cress
salt

Directions

To begin, mix together the maple syrup, soy sauce and lime juice to make the glaze. Set 6 tablespoons aside for the vegetables
Place the 4 salmon fillets in a tray and pour over the remaining glaze. Leave the salmon to marinate for 20 minutes
To prepare the vegetables, cut the white and green asparagus into 3cm batons. Bring a large pan of salted water to the boil and drop in the green asparagus. 1 minute later drop in the white, then a minute later the wild asparagus, peas and broad beans

Leave to cook for an additional 2 minutes, then drain and refresh in ice cold water for 5 minutes. Drain again and refrigerate until required

Preheat the oven to 160°C/gas mark 3

Place a non-stick pan over a high heat and add a tiny drop of vegetable oil. Remove the salmon from the marinade and allow any excess to drip off

Add the salmon pieces to the pan and quickly sear all over – the glaze will burn if you leave the fish in the pan too long, so take care. Clean the pan, then repeat with the remaining 2 fillets

Once the salmon has a caramelised brown colour, transfer to a baking tray and place in the oven until it is cooked to the desired temperature – slightly pink in the middle is ideal and will take 3–6 minutes depending on the thickness of the fillets. Leave to cook for longer if desired

Warm the blanched vegetables quickly in a pan with a dash of oil and place them in a bowl. Drizzle a little of the reserved marinade over them and add the salad leaves and coriander

Divide the vegetables between serving bowls and arrange the salmon fillets on top. Sprinkle with the toasted sesame seeds and serve immediately

Crunchy Crunch

Servings:

12

Yield:

2 dozen

Ingredients

2 cups butterscotch chips

¼ cup peanut butter

3 ½ cups cornflakes cereal

Directions

1

Melt the butterscotch chips over low heat and add peanut butter.

2

Stir in cornflakes.

3

Drop on waxed paper and let cool.

Nutritions

Per Serving: 223 calories; protein 1.9g; carbohydrates 26.4g; fat 10.8g; sodium 114mg.

Jamaica Cake

Servings:
14
Yield:
1 - 13x9 inch pan

Ingredients

2 cups white sugar

1 ½ cups vegetable oil

1 ½ cups chopped pecans

3 cups all-purpose flour

2 bananas, peeled and diced

3 eggs

1 (20 ounce) can crushed pineapple with juice

1 teaspoon vanilla extract

1 teaspoon salt

1 teaspoon baking soda

Directions
   1

Mix together sugar, vegetable oil, pecans, flour, and bananas in a 13 x 9 inch pan. Stir in the eggs, pineapple (with juice), vanilla, salt and baking soda. Mix well. Do not mash the bananas.

   2

Bake in a preheated 350 degrees F (175 degrees C) oven for 60 minutes or until cake tests done.

Nutritions

Per Serving: 552 calories; protein 5.5g; carbohydrates 60.9g; fat 33.4g; cholesterol 39.9mg; sodium 272.1mg.

Apricot Acid

Servings:

6

Yield:

6 servings

Ingredients

3 (15 ounce) cans apricot halves, drained

¾ cup packed brown sugar

50 buttery round crackers, crumbled

½ cup butter, melted

Directions

1

Preheat oven to 325 degrees F (165 degrees C).

2

In an 8x12 inch baking pan, layer half of apricots, brown sugar, cracker crumbs, and butter. Repeat.

3

Bake for 50 to 60 minutes.

Nutritions

Per Serving: 588 calories; protein 3.4g; carbohydrates 100g; fat 21.7g; cholesterol 61.5mg; sodium 341.9mg.

Beetroot Hummus

Prep:

25 mins

Cook:

1 hr 20 mins

Additional:

12 hrs

Total:

13 hrs 45 mins

Servings:

8

Yield:

8 servings

Ingredients

8 ounces chickpeas

1 large onion, chopped

1 pound beets

½ cup tahini

3 cloves garlic, crushed

¼ cup fresh lemon juice

1 tablespoon ground cumin

¼ cup olive oil

Directions

1

In a large bowl, cover chickpeas with cold water and soak overnight.

2

Drain chickpeas and place in a large heavy saucepan; add onion, cover with water and bring to a boil over medium heat. Cook for 1 hour, or until chickpeas are very soft. Drain, reserving 1 cup of cooking liquid. Allow to cool.

3

Meanwhile, in a large saucepan cover beets with water and bring to a boil over medium heat. Cook until tender; drain and allow beets to cool before removing the skins and chopping.

4

Puree beets in a food processor; add the chickpeas and onions, tahini, garlic, lemon juice and cumin. Process until smooth. Slowly, while the machine is running, pour in the reserved cooking liquid and olive oil. Continue to process until mixture is thoroughly combined. Drizzle with a little olive oil.

Nutritions

Per Serving: 219 calories; protein 5.3g; carbohydrates 17.8g; fat 15.4g; sodium 142.3mg.

Chicken Tacos

Prep:

15 mins

Cook:

40 mins

Total:

55 mins

Servings:

8

Yield:

8 tacos

Ingredients

¼ cup water

1 (1 ounce) packet taco seasoning mix

2 (8 ounce) cans tomato sauce

2 teaspoons white distilled vinegar

2 teaspoons minced garlic

2 teaspoons ground oregano

1 teaspoon ground cumin

½ teaspoon white sugar

2 tablespoons olive oil

2 pounds skinless, boneless chicken breasts

8 taco shells, warmed

Directions

1

Mix water and taco seasoning in a large bowl. Add tomato sauce, vinegar, garlic, oregano, cumin, and sugar; mix well.

2

Heat oil in a large skillet over medium-high heat. Add chicken and cook until golden brown, about 5 minutes per side. Add tomato sauce mixture and bring to a boil. Reduce heat to medium-low, cover, and simmer until chicken is no longer pink in the center and the juices run clear, about 20 minutes. An instant-read thermometer inserted into the center should read at least 165 degrees F (74 degrees C).

3

Remove chicken breasts from the pan and shred meat with 2 forks when cool enough to handle. Return shredded chicken to the pan with the tomato sauce. Cook and stir until chicken is coated with sauce and sauce reduces a bit, about 5 minutes.

4

Transfer chicken and sauce to a serving bowl and spoon onto taco shells.

Nutritions

Per Serving: 244 calories; protein 24g; carbohydrates 15.7g; fat 9g; cholesterol 58.5mg; sodium 658.8mg.

Veggie Chili

Prep:
45 mins

Cook:
1 hr

Total:
1 hr 45 mins

Servings:
8

Yield:
8 servings

Ingredients

½ cup texturized vegetable protein (TVP)

1 cup water

2 ½ tablespoons olive oil

1 onion, chopped

6 cloves garlic, minced

1 teaspoon salt

1 teaspoon ground black pepper

2 teaspoons chili powder

2 teaspoons ground cumin

2 teaspoons ground cayenne pepper

¼ teaspoon cinnamon

1 tablespoon honey

2 (12 ounce) cans kidney beans with liquid

2 (12 ounce) cans diced tomatoes with juice

1 green bell pepper, chopped

2 carrots, finely chopped

1 bunch green onions, chopped

1 bunch cilantro, chopped

1 (8 ounce) container dairy sour cream

Directions

1

Place the textured vegetable protein (TVP) in water, and soak 30 minutes. Press to drain.

2

Heat the oil in a large pot over medium heat, and saute TVP, onion, and garlic until onion is tender and TVP is evenly browned. Season with salt, pepper, 1/2 the chili powder, 1/2 the cumin, 1/2 the cayenne pepper, and cinnamon. Mix in honey, beans, tomatoes, green bell pepper, and carrots. Cook, stirring, occasionally, 45 minutes.

3

Season the chili with remaining chili powder, cumin, and cayenne pepper, and continue cooking 15 minutes. To serve, divide into bowls, garnish with green onions and cilantro, and top with dollops of sour cream.

Nutritions

Per Serving: 253 calories; protein 13.3g; carbohydrates 27.2g; fat 11.2g; cholesterol 12.5mg; sodium 718.4mg.

CHAPTER 5: DINNER

Salad with Brie and Apple

Prep:10 mins
Total:10 mins
Servings:4

Ingredients

½ cup balsamic vinaigrette
½ cup sliced Brie cheese
3 cups spring mix salad greens
2 red apples, cored and thinly sliced
⅓ cup toasted walnut pieces

Directions

Toss the apple slices with the vinaigrette in a bowl until evenly coated;
add the greens and toss again; top with the Brie and walnuts just
before serving.

Nutrition

:
258 calories; protein 6.1g; carbohydrates 15.2g; fat 20.7g; cholesterol
18mg; sodium 474.6mg.

Turmeric Scallops

Serves 4 (serving size 4 large scallops)

Ingredients:

16 large wild-caught sea scallops (10-20 size, about 1 1/2 pounds)
1 Tablespoon coconut oil
1/3 bunch of parsley, leaves only, finely chopped
6-8 large cloves garlic, minced
1 Tablespoon ground turmeric
1 1/2 teaspoons kosher salt
1/4 cup extra-virgin olive oil

Directions

In medium to large bowl mix garlic, parsley, turmeric, olive oil, and
salt. Next add scallops and toss to coat. Be sure to use tongs or gloved
hands, to avoid turning your fingers yellow from the turmeric.
Heat skillet to medium-high heat and add coconut oil. When oil is hot
add scallops. Cook approximately 2 minutes per side or until scallops
are opaque and feel slightly firm to the touch. Be careful not to
overcook as it will result in the scallops being tough.
Serve over a salad of mixed greens with a light vinaigrette - in this case
used mache greens with a blood orange and citrus champagne
vinaigrette (juice from blood oranges, citrus champagne vinegar, thinly
sliced green onion-whites only, minced garlic, EVOO, kosher salt).

Balsamic Beet Salad

Prep Time: 15 minutes
Cook Time: 15 minutes (Instant Pot timing)

INGREDIENTS

4 medium beets
1 recipe Best Balsamic Vinaigrette
2 ounces soft goat cheese
5 ounces baby arugula or baby green
1/4 cup roasted salted pistachios, roughly chopped

DIRECTIONS

Cook the beets: Use our Oven Roasted Beets or Instant Pot
Beets method.
Slice the beets: Slice the beets into wedges. Take proper precautions as
beet juice stains easily).
Make the dressing: In a medium bowl, make the Best Balsamic
Vinaigrette.
Toss the beets with the dressing (optional): Place the beets in the bowl
with the dressing and stir. The beets will change the color of the
dressing to a bright pink color and infuse a little sweetness. If you'd
rather keep the balsamic vinaigrette color, you can skip this s.
Assemble the salad: Thinly slice the shallot. Place the greens on a plate.
Remove the beets from the dressing bowl and place them on top. Add
crumbles of goat cheese, shallot, and chopped pistachios. Drizzle with
dressing and serve.

Nutritions

Total Fat 8g

145

6%Total Carbohydrate 16.4g

14%Dietary Fiber 4g

Sugars 10.7g

14%Protein 7.1g

26%Vitamin A 237.3µg

17%Vitamin C 15.2mg

8%Calcium 108.8mg

13%Iron 2.3mg

1%Vitamin D 0.1µg

15%Magnesium 64.4mg

Egg White Pizza

Serves 1
Prep: 10 mins
Cook: About 40 Mins

Ingredients

9 T liquid egg whites (about 4 large egg whites)
2 T pizza sauce (I just used generic store bought)
1/3 C mozzarella cheese
1/2 serving turkey pepperoni
2-3 sliced muchrooms
1 serving black olives sliced
1/4 C sliced sweet pepper

Directions

Slice mushrooms, olives, and peppers thin and have ready to go.
Heat a medium sized non stick frying pan to medium heat and spray good with nonstick spray.
When pan is warm, pour in egg whites and sprinkle some salt and pepper on. It's also good to sprinkle a little garlic salt in place of salt if you like.
Let eggs cook until just starting to set. It needs to get to the point that you can flip the whole thing over without messing it up too much.
When the eggs are ready carefully flip over in the pan and take off the heat while you quickly add the toppings on the cooked side like you would making a pizza.
Turn the heat down to low, cover with a lid and put the pan back on the heat until the cheese is all melted.
One option would be to sautee your veggies ahead of time of you want them more cooked. I like them still kind of crisp but warm, but it's all up to your preference.

Oxtail Soup

Prep:20 mins
Cook:12 hrs 10 mins
Additional:1 hr
Servings:8

Ingredients

2 tablespoons butter
1 onion, chopped
½ (750 milliliter) bottle red wine
1 pound beef oxtail, cut into pieces
water to cover
salt and ground black pepper to taste
1 pound potatoes, peeled and cubed
2 ribs celery, chopped
1 cup green beans
2 carrots, chopped
1 (14.5 ounce) can stewed tomatoes

Directions

Heat butter in a large skillet over medium heat. Add oxtail and onion; cook until oxtail is until browned, 6 to 7 minutes per side. Transfer oxtail and onion to a slow cooker.
Pour wine into the skillet and bring to a boil while scraping the browned bits of food off the bottom of the skillet with a wooden spoon. Pour wine mixture into slow cooker; add water to cover.
Set slow cooker to Low; cook soup for 8 hours. Add potatoes, carrots, celery, and green beans; cook soup for 4 hours more.

Cool soup slightly; refrigerate until fat has risen to top and solidified, about 1 hour. Scoop off fat; stir in tomatoes. Reheat soup on stove before serving.

Nutrition

211 calories; protein 11g; carbohydrates 18.7g; fat 6.9g; cholesterol 38.8mg; sodium 241.3mg.

Linguine Shrimps & Garlic

Prep:10 mins
Cook:20 mins
Servings:4

Ingredients

1 (16 ounce) package fresh linguine pasta
1 pound large shrimp, peeled and deveined
3 tablespoons chopped fresh basil
3 tablespoons olive oil, divided
 tablespoons butter, cut up
¼ cup grated Asiago cheese
2 teaspoons minced garlic

Directions

Bring a large pot of lightly salted water and 1 tablespoon oil to a boil.
Cook linguine in the boiling water, stirring occasionally, until tender
yet firm to the bite, about 8 minutes. Drain and set aside.
Heat remaining olive oil in a large skillet over medium-high heat. Add
shrimp and saute until shrimp turns pink, 3 to 4 minutes. Add basil
and garlic; cook for 2 to 3 minutes more.
Add butter and cooked linguine. Toss until butter melts, making sure
to coat the linguine with the sauce. Remove from heat. Serve
immediately.

Nutrition

729 calories; protein 33.5g; carbohydrates 72g; fat 34.2g; cholesterol
267.3mg; sodium 477.4mg.

Mediterranean Vegetable Soup

Prep Time: 15 mins
Cook Time: 30 mins
Yield: Serves up to 6

INGREDIENTS

8 oz sliced baby bella mushrooms
1 bunch flat leaf parsley, washed, dried, stems and leaves separated, then each chopped
1 medium-size yellow or red onion, chopped
2 garlic cloves, chopped
Extra Virgin Olive oil
2 celery ribs, chopped
2 medium zucchini, tops removed, sliced into rounds or half-moons or diced
2 carrots, peeled, chopped
1 tsp ground coriander
½ tsp turmeric powder
½ tsp sweet paprika
2 golden potatoes, peeled, small diced
½ tsp dry thyme
1 32-oz can whole peeled tomatoes
1 15-oz can chickpeas, rinsed and drained
Salt and pepper
2 bay leaves
Zest of 1 lime
Juice of 1 lime
6 cups low-sodium vegetable or chicken broth

DIRECTIONS

In a large pot like this one (affiliate) heat 1 tbsp olive oil over medium-high until shimmering but not smoking. Add the mushrooms and cook for 3-5 minutes, stirring regularly. Remove from the pot and set aside from now.

Add more olive oil, if needed and heat. Add the chopped
parsley stems (stems only at this point), onions, garlic, celery, carrots, zucchini and small diced potatoes. Stir in the spices, and season with salt and pepper. Cook for about 7 minutes, stirring regularly, until the vegetables have softened a bit.

Now add the chickpeas, tomatoes, bay leaves, and broth. Bring to a boil for 5 minutes, then turn the heat down to medium-low. Cover only partway and cook for 15 more minutes.

Uncover and add the sauteed mushrooms. Cook for just a few more minutes until mushrooms are warmed through.

Finally, stir in the parsley leaves, lime zest, and lime juice.

Remove from the heat. Remove bay leaves. Transfer the vegetable soup to serving bowls and top with toasted pine nuts, if you like. Add a side of your favorite crusty bread or pita along with extra lime wedges and crushed red pepper. Enjoy!

Alfredo Sauce Pasta

Prep:5 mins
Cook:5 mins
Servings:4

Ingredients

1 (8 ounce) package cream cheese
2 teaspoons garlic powder
2 cups milk
6 ounces grated Parmesan cheese
½ cup butter
⅛ teaspoon ground black pepper

Directions

Melt butter in a medium, non-stick saucepan over medium heat. Add cream cheese and garlic powder, stirring with wire whisk until smooth. Add milk, a little at a time, whisking to smooth out lumps. Stir in Parmesan and pepper. Remove from heat when sauce reaches desired consistency. Sauce will thicken rapidly, thin with milk if cooked too long. Toss with hot pasta to serve.

Nutrition

648 calories; protein 25.1g; carbohydrates 10g; fat 57.1g; cholesterol 169.8mg; sodium 1029.8mg.

Salsa Jalapeno

Prep:15 mins
Cook:12 mins
Servings:25

Ingredients

10 fresh jalapeno peppers
1 white onion, quartered
¼ cup chopped fresh cilantro, or more to taste
2 cloves garlic, smashed
1 lime, juiced
2 tomatoes
1 teaspoon ground black pepper
1 teaspoon salt

Directions

Place jalapenos in a saucepan with enough water to cover. Bring to a boil. Simmer until jalapenos soften and begin to lose their shine, about 10 to 12 minutes. Remove the jalapenos with a slotted spoon, chop off the stem, and place them in a blender. Add the tomatoes and boil for 2 to 3 minutes to loosen the skin. Peel the skin from the tomatoes and add tomatoes to the blender.
Place the onion, cilantro, garlic, lime juice, salt, and black pepper in the blender with the jalapenos and tomatoes. Blend to desired consistency.

Nutrition

7 calories; protein 0.3g; carbohydrates 1.6g; fat 0.1g; sodium 94.1mg

Italian Seasoning Chicken

Prep:20 mins
Cook:1 hr 10 mins
Servings:6

Ingredients

4 large links hot Italian sausage
6 bone-in, skin on chicken thighs
1 small red onion, sliced
2 tablespoons olive oil, divided
½ yellow onion, sliced
4 large Yukon Gold potatoes, quartered
½ pound assorted sweet peppers, seeded
2 teaspoons dried Italian herbs
Freshly ground black pepper to taste
1 tablespoon Chopped fresh Italian parsley
2 teaspoons kosher salt, plus more as needed

Directions

Heat olive oil in a skillet over medium heat. Cook sausage links until browned and oil begins to render, about 3 minutes per side. While sausages are cooking, pierce them lightly here and there with the tip of a sharp knife so some fats and juices are released. Remove from heat and let cool slightly.

When sausages are cool enough to handle, cut them into serving pieces, about 2-inch slices. Transfer back to pan along with any accumulated juices from the cutting board.

Cut two slashes down to the bone on the skin side of each chicken thigh.

Depending on the size of the peppers, halve or quarter them and place in a large mixing bowl. Add the sliced red and yellow onions and potato chunks. Add chicken thighs and sausage pieces with pan juices. Season with kosher salt, black pepper, and Italian herbs. Drizzle with a tablespoon of olive oil.

Mix with your hands until all ingredients are coated in oil, 3 or 4 minutes. Transfer to large, heavy-duty roasting pan. Evenly space the chicken thighs skin side up. Position potatoes near the top.

Place in preheated oven until chicken is cooked through and everything is caramelized, about 1 hour. An instant-read thermometer inserted near the bone should read 165 degrees F. Sprinkle with chopped fresh Italian parsley, if desired.

Scampi Linguini

Prep:25 mins
Cook:20 mins
Servings:4

Ingredients

1 (16 ounce) package linguine
¼ cup butter
6 cloves garlic, minced
1 pound peeled and deveined medium shrimp
¾ cup white wine
¼ cup olive oil
¼ teaspoon crushed red pepper
1 tablespoon chopped fresh basil
½ teaspoon salt
½ cup lemon juice
½ pint grape tomatoes, halved
1 tablespoon chopped fresh parsley
2 tablespoons grated Pecorino Romano cheese

Directions

Fill a large pot with lightly salted water and bring to a rolling boil over high heat. Once the water is boiling, stir in the linguine, and return to a boil. Cook the pasta uncovered, stirring occasionally, until the pasta has cooked through, but is still firm to the bite, about 12 minutes. Drain well in a colander set in the sink. Transfer the linguine to a large mixing bowl.

Heat the olive oil and butter together in large skillet over medium heat until the butter is melted. Cook and stir the garlic in the butter and oil for 3 minutes. Add shrimp and cook for 5 minutes, stirring frequently. Stir in the wine, lemon juice, red pepper, basil, and salt and cook another 1 minute. Mix in the tomatoes and cook 1 minute more; remove from heat and transfer mixture to the bowl with the linguine. Sprinkle the Pecorino Romano cheese and parsley over the pasta and sauce; toss until well mixed.

Nutrition

707 calories; protein 33.3g; carbohydrates 68.6g; fat 29.7g; cholesterol 288.7mg; sodium 652mg.

Pad Thai

Prep:40 mins
Cook:20 mins
Servings:6

Ingredients

2 tablespoons butter
1 pound boneless, skinless chicken breast halves, cut into bite-sized pieces
¼ cup vegetable oil
4 eggs
1 (12 ounce) package rice noodles
2 tablespoons fish sauce
3 tablespoons white sugar
1 tablespoon white wine vinegar
2 cups bean sprouts
¼ cup crushed peanuts
⅛ tablespoon crushed red pepper
1 lemon, cut into wedges
3 green onions, chopped

Directions

Soak rice noodles in cold water 35 to 50 minutes, or until soft. Drain, and set aside.
Heat butter in a wok or large heavy skillet. Saute chicken until browned. Remove, and set aside. Heat oil in wok over medium-high heat. Crack eggs into hot oil, and cook until firm. Stir in chicken, and cook for 5 minutes. Add softened noodles, and vinegar, fish sauce, sugar and red pepper. Adjust seasonings to taste. Mix while cooking, until noodles are tender. Add bean sprouts, and mix for 3 minutes.

Nutrition

524 calories; protein 26.4g; carbohydrates 58.5g; fat 20.7g; cholesterol 178.1mg; sodium 593.6mg.

Jamaican Curried Goat

Prep:15 mins
Cook:1 hr 44 mins
Additional:1 hr
Servings:8

Ingredients

2 pounds goat stew meat, cut into 1-inch cubes
2 tablespoons curry powder
2 cloves garlic, minced
2 fresh hot chile peppers, seeded and chopped
1 teaspoon salt
3 tablespoons vegetable oil
1 onion, chopped
1 teaspoon ground black pepper
1 rib celery, chopped
2 ½ cups vegetable broth
3 potatoes, peeled and cut into 1-inch chunks
1 bay leaf

Directions

Combine goat meat, chile pepper, curry powder, garlic, salt, and black pepper in a bowl. Cover and refrigerate to allow flavors to blend, 1 hour to overnight.

Remove goat meat mixture from bowl and pat dry, reserving marinade. Heat vegetable oil in a stockpot over medium-high heat. Cook meat in batches, browning on all sides, 4 to 6 minutes per batch. Transfer meat to a plate. Add onion and celery to the stockpot; cook and stir until onion begins to brown, 4 to 6 minutes.

Stir browned goat meat into onion mixture. Add reserved marinade, vegetable broth, and bay leaf. Bring to a boil, cover, reduce heat to low, and simmer for 1 hour. Stir in potatoes; simmer until potatoes and meat are tender, 35 to 45 minutes more.

Remove stockpot from heat, skim off surface fat, and remove bay leaf.

Nutrition

238 calories; protein 21.9g; carbohydrates 20.1g; fat 7.8g; cholesterol 53.2mg; sodium 509.3mg.

Crab Stew

Serves 6

Ingredients

12 large live blue crabs
½ cup all-purpose flour
1¼ cups chopped onion
¼ cup vegetable oil
¼ cup chopped green bell pepper
¾ cup chopped celery
2 bay leaves
¼ cup chopped red bell pepper
1 teaspoon salt
6 cups seafood stock
1 pound lump crabmeat, picked free of shells
½ teaspoon cayenne pepper
1½ pounds large fresh shrimp, peeled and deveined
2 tablespoons finely chopped fresh parsley

Directions

Scald crabs with hot water to stun. Remove the back sep (top shell) from each crab, and clean out gills, lungs, and center of each. Crack crabs in half, and remove claws. Reserve claws for stock.
In a large heavy stockpot, combine oil and flour, and heat over medium heat. Stirring slowly, make a dark-brown roux, 15 to 20 minutes. Add onion, bell peppers, and celery. Cook, stirring frequently, until vegetables are soft, about 5 minutes. Add bay leaves, salt, cayenne, and seafood stock. Stir to combine. Bring mixture to a boil over high heat; reduce heat to medium-low, add crabs, and simmer 20 minutes. Add crabmeat and shrimp, and cook 10 minutes. Remove from heat, and add parsley. Serve hot.

Lime Lobsters

Serves: 4 People
Prep time: 15m
Cook Time: 10m

Ingredients

4 Lobster tails (6-7 oz.)
1/2 Teaspoon Paprika
2 Tablespoons Lime Juice
1 Tablespoon Olive Oil
2 Tablespoons Butter

Directions

Rinse lobster tails: pat dry with paper towels. Use kitchen sheers to cut through hard top shell of lobster tail, cutting through meat, but not through the lower shell. Spread meat open in shell. Preheat broiler. In a small bowl whisk together butter, like juice, olive oil and paprika. Place lobster tails, meat size up, on the broiler pan rack. Set aside 3 tablespoons of butter mixture; keep warm. Brush lobster meat with remaining butter mixture.
Broil 4 to 5 inches from heat for 6 minutes or until opaque in center. Be careful NOT to overcook. Drizzle with reserved butter mixture.

Chili Mussels

0:30 Prep
0:25 Cook
4 Servings

INGREDIENTS

2 tablespoons olive oil
2 garlic cloves, crushed
2 small red chillies, deseeded, finely chopped
1 brown onion, finely chopped
1 tablespoon tomato paste
1 lemon, rind finely grated, juiced
2 teaspoons caster sugar
1kg tomatoes, finely chopped
1/2 cup dry white wine
1.5kg mussels, beards removed
1/2 cup flat-leaf parsley leaves, roughly chopped
Salt and pepper, to season
Crusty bread, to serve

Directions

Heat oil in a large, deep saucepan over medium heat. Add onion, garlic and chilli. Cook, stirring, for 3 minutes or until onion is soft. Add tomato paste and cook for 1 minute.

Add tomato, lemon rind, lemon juice, sugar and wine to pan. Stir until well combined. Increase heat to high. Bring sauce to the boil. Reduce heat to medium. Simmer, uncovered, for 8 to 10 minutes or until thick. Season with salt and pepper.

Add mussels to sauce. Cover and cook, shaking pan occasionally, for 4 to 6 minutes or until mussel shells open. Discard unopened shells.

Ladle sauce and mussels into bowls. Sprinkle with parsley. Serve with bread.

Nutritions

1019 kj
Fat 2g
Fiber 18g
Proteing 23mg

Seafood Gratin

Prep:20 mins
Cook:1 hr
Servings:8

Ingredients

1 green bell pepper, chopped
1 cup butter, divided
1 pound fresh crabmeat
1 onion, chopper
4 cups water
1 pound fresh shrimp, peeled and deveined
1 cup all-purpose flour, divided
½ pound small scallops
½ pound flounder fillets
1 cup shredded sharp Cheddar cheese
1 tablespoon distilled white vinegar
3 cups milk
1 teaspoon Worcestershire sauce
½ teaspoon salt
1 dash hot pepper sauce
½ cup grated Parmesan cheese
1 pinch ground black pepper

Directions

In a heavy skillet, saute the onion and the pepper in 1/2 cup of butter.
Cook until tender. Mix in 1/2 cup of the flour, and cook over medium
heat for 10 minutes, stirring frequently. Stir in crabmeat, remove from
heat, and set aside.

In a large Dutch oven, bring the water to a boil. Add the shrimp, scallops, and flounder, and simmer for 3 minutes. Drain, reserving 1 cup of the cooking liquid, and set the seafood aside.

In a heavy saucepan, melt the remaining 1/2 cup butter over low heat. Stir in remaining 1/2 cup flour. Cook and stir constantly for 1 minute. Gradually add the milk plus the 1 cup reserved cooking liquid. Raise heat to medium; cook, stirring constantly, until the mixture is thickened and bubbly. Mix in the shredded Cheddar cheese, vinegar, Worcestershire sauce, salt, pepper, and hot sauce. Stir in cooked seafood.

Preheat oven to 350 degrees F . Lightly grease one 9x13 inch baking dish. Press crabmeat mixture into the bottom of the prepared pan. Spoon the seafood mixture over the crabmeat crust, and sprinkle with the Parmesan cheese.

Bake in the preheated oven for 30 minutes, or until lightly browned. Serve immediately.

Nutrition

66 calories; protein 42.8g; carbohydrates 20.4g; fat 34.2g; cholesterol 233.3mg; sodium 858.9mg.

Sri Lanka Vegetarian Curry

45 Minutes

Serves 4

Ingredients

oil for frying

garlic 2 cloves, sliced

green chillies 3, sliced

Sri Lankan curry powder 2 tbsp (see below)

turmeric 1 tsp

onions 2, halved and sliced

black mustard seeds 1 tsp

coconut milk 400g tin

butternut squash 200g, cubed

cauliflower 1 small, broken into small florets

vegetable stock 200ml

runner beans 100g, trimmed and sliced

curry leaves 10

steamed rice to serve

SRI LANKAN CURRY POWDER

coriander seeds 2 tsp

cumin seeds 1 tsp

star anise 1/2

cinnamon ½ stick broken

cloves 6

cardamom 2 pods

black peppercorns ½ tsp

fennel seeds 1 tsp

fenugreek ½ tsp

small dried red chillis 3-5 (depending on how hot you like it)

basmati or jasmine rice 1 tbsp

Directions

To make the curry powder, dry-fry the spices and chilli in a non-stick frying pan until fragrant and darkened a little. Tip out
of the pan and cool. Add the rice to the pan and dry-fry until pale golden. Cool. Tip everything into a spice or coffee grinder and whizz to a powder.

Heat 3 tbsp oil in a large pan. Add the onions and cook until soft and golden, about 10 minutes. Add the garlic and chilli and cook for 3 minutes, then stir in 2 tbsp of the curry powder and turmeric and keep stirring until you start to smell the spices.

Add the coconut milk and stock and bring to a simmer. Drop in the squash, cook for 4-5 minutes, then add the cauli and cook for 3-4 minutes. Add the beans and cook until just tender.

To serve, heat another 2 tbsp of oil in a pan and fry the curry leaves and mustard seeds until they frazzle and begin to pop. Pour over the curry and serve wi

Bamboo Shoots Soup

Prep:10 mins
Cook:23 mins
Additional:15 mins
Servings:2

Ingredients

2 small dried cloud ear mushrooms
1 ½ cups water
4 ounces pork fillet, thinly sliced
2 tablespoons white sugar
2 tablespoons sake (Japanese rice wine)
2 tablespoons soy sauce
4 ounces canned bamboo shoots, drained and chopped
2 tablespoons black rice vinegar
3 eggs
1 ½ teaspoons sesame oil
1 teaspoon chile paste

Directions

Place mushrooms in a small bowl and cover with water. Let soak until softened, about 15 minutes. Drain and cut into bite-size pieces.
Bring 1 1/2 cup water to a boil in a pot. Add pork and bamboo shots. Cook, skimming off any fat that rises to the top, until pork is tender, 7 to 10 minutes.
Mix sugar, sake, soy sauce, black rice vinegar, and chile paste together in a small bowl. Stir into the pot. Reduce heat to low and simmer soup, covered, about 10 minutes.
Stir mushroom pieces into the soup. Crack in eggs and cook, covered, until whites are firm and the yolks have thickened but are not hard, 2 to 3 minutes. Drizzle sesame oil over soup before serving.

Nutrition

323 calories; protein 21.4g; carbohydrates 23.9g; fat 14.7g; cholesterol 305.1mg; sodium 1059.8mg.

Chicken with Green Onion Sauce

Prep:6 mins
Cook:27 mins
Yield:4 servings (serving size: 1 chicken breast half)

Ingredients

2 tablespoons all-purpose flour
2 garlic cloves, minced
¼ teaspoon dried thyme
1 (14-ounce) can fat-free, less-sodium chicken broth
Cooking spray
⅓ cup finely chopped green onions, divided
⅛ teaspoon salt
4 (4-ounce) skinless, boneless chicken breast halves
⅛ teaspoon pepper

Directions

1Combine 1/4 cup broth and flour in a small bowl, stirring with a whisk until smooth. Add remaining broth, garlic, and thyme; set aside. Place a large nonstick skillet coated with cooking spray over medium-high heat until hot. Add chicken, and cook 4 to 5 minutes or until lightly browned. Turn chicken; add 2 tablespoons green onions. Pour broth mixture over chicken; sprinkle with salt and pepper. Reduce heat, and simmer, uncovered, 17 to 20 minutes or until chicken is done, basting often.
Remove chicken from pan; keep warm. Bring sauce to a boil over medium-high heat. Scrape bottom and sides of pan, using a rubber spatula. Cook 2 minutes or until sauce is reduced to 3/4 cup. Pour sauce evenly over chicken, and top with remaining green onions.

Nutrition

155 calories; fat 2.1g; saturated fat 0.7g; protein 28g; carbohydrates 4.3g; cholesterol 67mg; iron 1.1mg; sodium 195mg; calories from fat 13%; fiber 0.2g; calcium 24mg.

Shredded Chicken

Prep:5 mins
Cook:3 hrs
Servings:12

Ingredients

1 cup chicken broth
½ teaspoon seasoned salt, or to taste
3 pounds skinless, boneless chicken breast halves

Directions

Place chicken breasts in the bottom of a slow cooker. Pour in chicken broth and seasoned salt. Cover and cook on High until no longer pink in the center and the juices run clear, 3 to 4 hours, or on Low for 6 to 8 hours. An instant-read thermometer inserted into the center of the chicken breasts should read at least 165 degrees F .
Remove chicken and shred with 2 forks.

Beef Brisket

Prep:15 mins
Cook:6 hrs 15 mins
Servings:6

Ingredients

1 (5 pound) flat-cut corned beef brisket
2 tablespoons water
1 tablespoon browning sauce (such as Kitchen Bouquet®), or as desired
1 tablespoon vegetable oil
6 cloves garlic, sliced
1 onion, sliced

Directions

Preheat oven to 275 degrees F .
Discard any flavoring packet from corned beef. Brush brisket with browning sauce on both sides. Heat vegetable oil in a large skillet over medium-high heat and brown brisket on both sides in the hot oil, 6 to 8 minutes per side.
Place brisket on a rack set in a roasting pan. Scatter onion and garlic slices over brisket and add water to roasting pan. Cover pan tightly with aluminum foil.
Roast in the preheated oven until meat is tender, about 6 hours.

Nutrition

:
455 calories; protein 30.6g; carbohydrates 5.4g; fat 33.7g; cholesterol 162mg; sodium 1877.4mg.

Beef Chimicangas

Prep: 25 min. Cook: 15 min.
Makes 1 dozen

Ingredients

1 pound ground beef
1 can (16 ounces) refried beans
3 cans (8 ounces each) tomato sauce, divided
2 teaspoons chili powder
1 teaspoon minced garlic
1/2 cup finely chopped onion
1/2 teaspoon ground cumin
12 flour tortillas (10 inches), warmed
1 can (4 ounces) chopped jalapeno peppers
Oil for deep-fat frying
1-1/2 cups shredded cheddar cheese
1 can (4 ounces) chopped green chiles

Directions

In a large skillet, cook beef over medium heat until no longer pink; drain. Stir in the beans, onion, 1/2 cup tomato sauce, chili powder, garlic and cumin.
Spoon about 1/3 cup of beef mixture off-center on each tortilla. Fold edge nearest filling up and over to cover. Fold in both sides and roll up. Fasten with toothpicks. In a large saucepan, combine the chilies, peppers and remaining tomato sauce; heat through.
In an electric skillet or deep-fat fryer, heat 1 in. of oil to 375°. Fry the chimichangas for 1-1/2 to 2 minutes on each side or until browned. Drain on paper towels. Sprinkle with cheese. Serve with sauce.

Nutrition

1 chimichanga: 626 calories, 41g fat (9g saturated fat), 37mg cholesterol, 1094mg sodium, 46g carbohydrate (5g sugars, 6g fiber), 19g protein.

Quinoa Tabbouleh

Prep:15 mins
Cook:15 mins
Servings:4

Ingredients

2 cups water
1 pinch salt
¼ cup olive oil
½ teaspoon sea salt
1 cup quinoa
3 tomatoes, diced
1 cucumber, diced
2 bunches green onions, diced
¼ cup lemon juice
1 cup chopped fresh parsley
2 carrots, grated

Directions

In a saucepan bring water to a boil. Add quinoa and a pinch of salt. Reduce heat to low, cover and simmer for 15 minutes. Allow to cool to room temperature; fluff with a fork.
Meanwhile, in a large bowl, combine olive oil, sea salt, lemon juice, tomatoes, cucumber, green onions, carrots and parsley. Stir in cooled quinoa.

Nutrition

354 calories; protein 9.6g; carbohydrates 45.7g; fat 16.6g; sodium 324.7mg

Salmon Balls with Lentis

Yield people
Serving Size1 patty

Ingredients

8 ounces wild Alaskan salmon fillet or 1 (14 ounce) can salmon, well-drained
1 tablespoon canola oil
1 tablespoon extra virgin olive oil
1 egg slightly beaten
1/2 onion finely diced
1/4 cup red bell pepper diced
1/2 cup lentils cooked, drained well
1/2 cup whole wheat panko or whole wheat bread crumbs
1/2 teaspoon black pepper
1/2 teaspoon dried thyme
1/8 teaspoon cayenne pepper
kosher or sea salt to taste

Directions

Preheat oven to broil.
If using salmon fillet, line a rimmed cookie sheet with foil, place salmon on a cookie sheet, spread olive oil on both sides. Broil on both sides 5-6 minutes or until it reaches an internal temperature of 131 degrees. Allow to cool then remove the skin.
Place salmon in a medium mixing bowl and flake using a fork. Add egg, lentils, onion, bell pepper, Panko, and spices to salmon, mash either by hand or use a potato masher. Shape salmon into 4 patties. Or, use a large circular cookie cutter, pack and press salmon mixture to form patties.

Add canola oil to a large skillet, turn to medium heat, and cook patties on each side for about 5 minutes or until cooked through and lightly browned.

Serve salmon patties as a main dish or as a burger style sandwich with your favorite condiments.

Nutrition

Serving: 1patty | Calories: 312kcal | Carbohydrates: 26g | Protein: 22g | Fat: 14g | Saturated
Fat: 2g | Cholesterol: 93mg | Sodium: 101mg | Fiber: 5g | Sugar: 2g

Scallops and Brussels Sprouts

YIELD
Makes 4 servings

INGREDIENTS

10 ounces Brussels sprouts, trimmed and halved lengthwise
3 bacon slices (3 ounces), cut crosswise into 1/2-inch pieces
1/4 teaspoon salt
1 cup low-sodium chicken broth
3/4 teaspoon cornstarch
2 teaspoons fresh lemon juice
1/4 cup plus 2 teaspoons water
1 1/2 tablespoons unsalted butter
Pinch of sugar
12 large sea scallops (1 1/4 pounds), tough muscle removed from side
of each if necessary
2 teaspoons olive oil

PREPARATION

Blanch Brussels sprouts in a 3- to 4-quart saucepan of boiling salted
water , uncovered, 3 minutes, then drain.
Cook bacon in a 10-inch heavy skillet over moderate heat, turning over
occasionally, until crisp. Transfer bacon with a slotted spoon to a small
bowl and reserve bacon fat in another small bowl.
Add 1/4 cup broth and 1/4 cup water to skillet and bring to a simmer,
scraping up any brown bits. Add butter, salt, sugar, a pinch of pepper,
and Brussels sprouts and simmer, covered, 4 minutes. Remove lid and
cook over moderately high heat, stirring occasionally, until all liquid is
evaporated and Brussels sprouts are tender and golden brown, about 8
minutes more. Stir in bacon and remove from heat.

While Brussels sprouts are browning, pat scallops dry and season with salt and pepper. Heat oil with 2 teaspoons bacon fat in a 12-inch heavy skillet over moderately high heat until hot but not smoking, then sear scallops, turning over once, until golden brown and just cooked through, 4 to 6 minutes total. Transfer to a platter as cooked and keep warm, loosely covered with foil.

Pour off and discard any fat from skillet used to cook scallops. Add remaining 3/4 cup broth and simmer, stirring and scraping up any brown bits, 1 minute. Stir cornstarch into remaining 2 teaspoons water in a cup, then stir into sauce along with any scallop juices accumulated on platter. Simmer, stirring, 1 minute, then remove from heat and stir in lemon juice and salt and pepper to taste.

Serve Brussels sprouts topped with scallops and sauce.

Exotic Palabok

Prep:30 mins

Cook:1 hr

Additional:4 hrs 10 mins

Servings:8

Ingredients

For the Exotic Marinade:

⅓ cup plain yogurt

1 medium lime, zested and juiced

2 teaspoons kosher salt

1 teaspoon ground paprika

1 teaspoon ground cumin

½ teaspoon ground coriander

¼ teaspoon cayenne pepper

¼ teaspoon ground white pepper

¼ teaspoon ground cinnamon

¼ teaspoon ground allspice

1 (2 to 3 pound) whole chicken, cut into 8 pieces

¼ teaspoon ground cardamom

For the Rice:

1 pinch saffron

2 ¼ cups chicken broth, divided

2 tablespoons unsalted butter

1 ½ cups basmati rice

1 drizzle olive oil

1 teaspoon kosher salt

salt to taste

Directions

Add yogurt, lime zest and juice, salt, paprika, cumin, coriander, cayenne, white pepper, cardamom, cinnamon, and allspice for marinade to a large mixing bowl; whisk to combine.

Make one or two slits into each piece of dark chicken meat, down to the bone. Add chicken parts to the yogurt marinade and toss very thoroughly. Wrap in plastic wrap and marinate in the refrigerator for 4 to 8 hours.

Preheat the oven to 450 degrees F. Lightly grease a 9x13-inch casserole dish.

Grind saffron in a mortar with a pestle. Pour in 1/4 cup chicken broth and stir to combine.

Combine unsalted butter and salt in a saucepan; pour in remaining 2 cups chicken broth and chicken broth-saffron mixture. Bring to a boil over high heat. Add basmati rice and stir to combine. Reduce heat to low, cover tightly, and let simmer gently for exactly 15 minutes; do not disturb while cooking. Turn off the heat and let rest for 10 minutes.

While rice is still hot, transfer into the prepared casserole dish. Use a fork to fluff the rice while gently spreading into an even layer. Place the chicken pieces, skin-side up, on top of rice. Drizzle with olive oil and sprinkle with salt.

Roast in the center of the preheated oven until chicken is no longer pink in the centers and juices run clear, about 45 minutes. An instant-read thermometer inserted into the thickest part of the thigh, near the bone, should read 165 degrees F .

While chicken is in the oven, mix yogurt, garlic, green onions, mint, cilantro, salt, and water together for sauce. Reserve in the refrigerator until needed. Serve chicken and rice on a plate and top with sauce.

Nutrition

362 calories; protein 23.8g; carbohydrates 31.7g; fat 15.4g; cholesterol 71.5mg; sodium 1125.5mg.

185

Yucatan Soup

Cook Time2 hrs 30 mins
Total Time2 hrs 30 mins

Ingredients

For the Tortillas
lard (for frying)
1 package corn tortillas (sliced into strips)
For the Soup
1 white onion thinly sliced
3 limes
1 cup long-grain white rice
1 whole chicken (about 3 pounds)
To Serve
Jalapeños
Cotija cheese
limes
avocados

Directions

Line a plate with a paper towel or a cotton kitchen towel.
Set a cast-iron skillet over medium heat. Spoon enough lard into the skillet so that when it melts, it reaches about 1/2 inch up the side of the skillet, about 11/2 cups.
Once the fat melts completely and begins to shimmer in the skillet, test the oil by dropping a tortilla strip into the hot fat. If the tortilla sizzles immediately in the pan, crisping and turning a golden brown within about 30 seconds, the oil is ready. Working in batches, and taking care not to crowd the pan, fry the tortilla strips until crisp and golden brown. Using a slotted spoon, transfer the tortilla strips to the lined plate, and allow them to cool. Turn off the heat.

Place the whole chicken in a large stock pot. Pour enough water into the pot to cover the chicken by 2 inches. Bring the pot to a boil over medium-high heat, then immediately reduce the heat to medium-low and simmer, covered, for 2 hours, or until the chicken is cooked through and the meat shreds easily with a fork. Turn off the heat. Carefully remove the chicken from the pot, setting it on a platter to allow it to cool until it's comfortable enough to handle. Remove and discard the skin, pull the meat from the bone, and shred it with a fork. Strain the broth in the pot through a fine-mesh sieve into a pitcher or jar, discarding the solids. Wipe out the pot to remove any stray debris, and then return the strained broth and reserved chicken meat to the pot. Stir in the onion and rice and then bring to a simmer over medium heat. While the soup warms, juice one of the limes and then stir the juice into the soup pot. Continue cooking until the onion is soft and translucent and the chicken is warmed. While soup is cooking, finely chop the remaining 2 limes, peel and all.
Ladle into soup bowls and serve with the chopped lime, sliced jalapeño, crumbled Cotija cheese, sliced avocado, and tortilla strips.

Salmon Chowder

Prep:15 mins
Cook:30 mins
Servings:8

Ingredients

3 tablespoons butter
½ cup chopped celery
1 teaspoon garlic powder
2 cups diced potatoes
¾ cup chopped onion
2 cups chicken broth
1 teaspoon salt
1 teaspoon ground black pepper
2 carrots, diced
½ pound Cheddar cheese, shredded
1 teaspoon dried dill weed
1 (12 fluid ounce) can evaporated milk
1 (15 ounce) can creamed corn
2 (16 ounce) cans salmon

Directions

Melt butter in a large pot over medium heat. Saute onion, celery, and garlic powder until onions are tender. Stir in potatoes, carrots, broth, salt, pepper, and dill. Bring to a boil, and reduce heat. Cover, and simmer 20 minutes.

Stir in salmon, evaporated milk, corn, and cheese. Cook until heated through.

Nutrition

490 calories; protein 38.6g; carbohydrates 26.5g; fat 25.9g; cholesterol 104.2mg; sodium 1139.5mg.

Fish Taco

Prep:40 mins
Cook:20 mins
Servings:8

Ingredients

1 cup all-purpose flour

1 teaspoon baking powder

½ teaspoon salt

1 egg

2 tablespoons cornstarch

1 cup beer

½ cup plain yogurt

½ cup mayonnaise

1 lime, juiced

1 jalapeno pepper, minced

1 teaspoon minced capers

½ teaspoon ground cumin

½ teaspoon dried dill weed

1 teaspoon ground cayenne pepper

½ teaspoon dried oregano

1 quart oil for frying

1 pound cod fillets, cut into 2 to 3 ounce portions

½ medium head cabbage, finely shredded

1 (12 ounce) package corn tortillas

Directions

To make beer batter: In a large bowl, combine flour, cornstarch, baking powder, and salt. Blend egg and beer, then quickly stir into the flour mixture (don't worry about a few lumps).

To make white sauce: In a medium bowl, mix together yogurt and mayonnaise. Gradually stir in fresh lime juice until consistency is slightly runny. Season with jalapeno, capers, oregano, cumin, dill, and cayenne.

Heat oil in deep-fryer to 375 degrees F.

Dust fish pieces lightly with flour. Dip into beer batter, and fry until crisp and golden brown. Drain on paper towels. Lightly fry tortillas; not too crisp. To serve, place fried fish in a tortilla, and top with shredded cabbage, and white sauce.

Nutrition

409 calories; protein 17.3g; carbohydrates 43g; fat 18.8g; cholesterol 54.3mg; sodium 406.5mg.

Vegetarian Pasticcio

READY IN: 1hr 30mins
SERVES: 8

INGREDIENTS

1 1/2 cups cooked lentils (I'd use brown)
3 tablespoons olive oil
3 tablespoons butter
2 onions, finely chopped
1 large eggplant, chopped into small pieces (unpeeled)
1 -2 garlic clove, minced
1/2 - 1teaspoon cinnamon
1/2 – 1teaspoon oregano
salt and pepper, to taste
1medium tomatoes, peeled and chopped or (32 ounce) can chopped tomatoes, drained
8 ounces tomato paste
1/2 – 1 cup parmesan cheese, grated
16 ounces cooked macaroni
CUSTARD SAUCE
3 tablespoons butter
3 cups milk, heated
3 eggs, beaten
3 tablespoons flour

DIRECTIONS

Preheat oven to 400°F.
Heat olive oil and butter over medium heat in a large skillet.
Add onions, eggplant, garlic and seasonings. Cover and let saute, stirring occasionally for about 10 minutes.
Add tomatoes and lentils with a little liquid. Cook until very thick.

Stir in tomato paste and heat through. Adjust seasonings to taste. Butter a large casserole of oblong baking dish and layer half of the noodles across the bottom. Sprinkle one third of the parmesan over the noodles. Layer half of the sauce over noodles and parmesan.
Layer the remaining half of the noodles over the sauce, sprinkle with one third of the parmesan and cover with the remaining sauce. *You could refrigerate it at this point if you want to make it ahead of time.
Custard Sauce:.
Heat butter in a saucepan over low heat, stir in flour, and let roux cook a few minutes.
Pour in heated milk, stirring with a whisk.
Slowly whisk sauce into beaten eggs.
Pour sauce over entire casserole. It should drain through to the bottom and bind the whole thing together. If it sits on top, slide a butter knife in and out of the layers in a few places.
Sprinkle with remaining parmesan and cover.
Bake for 1 hour.
Serve very hot.

Chicken Stock

Prep:

30 mins

Cook:

2 hrs 15 mins

Total:

2 hrs 45 mins

Servings:

12

Yield:

12 cups

Ingredients

cooking spray

3 carrots, coarsely chopped

3 stalks celery, coarsely chopped

1 onion, coarsely chopped

3 cloves garlic, smashed, or more to taste

2 tablespoons olive oil, or as needed, divided

2 bone-in chicken parts

water as needed

3 sprigs fresh thyme, or to taste

salt and ground black pepper to taste

Directions

1

Preheat the oven to 450 degrees F (230 degrees C). Spray a large rimmed baking sheet with cooking spray.

2

195

Combine carrots, celery, onion, and garlic with 1 tablespoon olive oil in a bowl. Arrange mixture loosely onto the prepared sheet, making sure not to crowd, as the vegetables will then steam instead of roast.

3
Roast the vegetables in the preheated oven until browned and fragrant, 15 to 25 minutes.

4
While the vegetables are roasting, heat remaining oil in a large stockpot over medium-high heat. Brown chicken parts in the hot oil until golden but not burned, adding 1/4 cup water at a time as needed, allowing it to boil off as to have bits stuck on the bottom of pan, 7 to 10 minutes. Pour in 1 quart water.

5
Transfer roasted vegetables to the stockpot. Pour 1/2 cup water onto the baking sheet, scrape up any bits, and pour into the stockpot. Repeat if necessary.

6
Add thyme, salt, and pepper to the pot with 2 to 4 quarts of water, depending on the size of your pot. Reduce heat to low and let simmer for 2 to 3 hours. Taste and adjust seasoning.

7
Line a sieve with cheesecloth and strain broth into a large pot or bowl; broth should come out clear and golden. If not using immediately, let cool completely before pouring into Mason® jars and freezing until ready to use.

Nutritions
Per Serving: 78 calories; protein 3.6g; carbohydrates 5.8g; fat 4.9g; cholesterol 13.2mg; sodium 58.6mg.

Coconut Haddock

Prep:

20 mins

Cook:

18 mins

Total:

38 mins

Servings:

4

Yield:

4 servings

Ingredients

1 tablespoon olive oil

1 pound haddock, cut into cubes

¼ cup chopped red bell pepper

1 shallot, finely chopped

1 clove garlic, minced

1 (13.5 ounce) can full-fat coconut milk

2 teaspoons red curry paste

2 teaspoons curry powder

¾ teaspoon ground coriander

¾ teaspoon ground turmeric

2 cups baby spinach

1 cup shelled edamame

2 green onions, sliced

Directions

1

Heat olive oil in a large pot until very hot. Add haddock; cook until browned, about 3 minutes per side. Add red bell pepper, shallot, and garlic; cook and stir until shallot softens, about 3 minutes.

2

Pour coconut milk into the pot. Whisk in curry paste, curry powder, coriander, and turmeric. Reduce heat; simmer until coconut milk is reduced by 1/4, 6 to 7 minutes. Stir in spinach and edamame. Cook until spinach is wilted and edamame is heated through, 3 to 4 minutes. Sprinkle green onions over curry.

Nutritions

Per Serving: 345 calories; protein 25.5g; carbohydrates 8.2g; fat 26.5g; cholesterol 65.5mg; sodium 153.4mg.

Cabbage Pear Salad

Prep:

15 mins

Cook:

20 mins

Total:

35 mins

Servings:

4

Yield:

4 servings

Ingredients

1 pound savoy cabbage, stalk removed

2 tablespoons unsalted butter, or more as needed

2 shallots, finely chopped

1 teaspoon confectioners' sugar, or to taste

1 tablespoon creamed horseradish

½ cup heavy whipping cream

salt and freshly ground black pepper to taste

cayenne pepper to taste

freshly ground nutmeg to taste

2 ripe pears - peeled, cored, and cubed

Directions

1

Bring a large pot of lightly salted water to a boil. Add cabbage and briefly blanch, about 3 minutes. Drain and rinse under cold water to stop the cooking process. Shred leaves finely.

2

Melt butter in a pot over medium-low heat and cook shallots until soft and translucent, about 5 minutes. Dust with confectioners sugar. Add blanched cabbage and cook, stirring occasionally, over medium heat, for about 3 minutes. Stir in horseradish and cream and bring to a simmer. Season with salt, pepper, cayenne, and nutmeg. Add pears and cook until heated through, about 3 minutes. Serve immediately.

Nutritions

Per Serving: 265 calories; protein 3.8g; carbohydrates 28.5g; fat 17.1g; cholesterol 56mg; sodium 361.6mg.

Kale and Garlic Platter

Prep:

5 mins

Cook:

10 mins

Total:

15 mins

Servings:

4

Yield:

4 servings

Ingredients

1 bunch kale
2 tablespoons olive oil
4 cloves garlic, minced

Directions

1

Tear the kale leaves into bite-size pieces from the thick stems; discard the stems.

2

Heat the olive oil in a large pot over medium heat. Cook and stir the garlic in the hot oil until softened, about 2 minutes. Add the kale and continue cooking and stirring until the kale is bright green and wilted, about 5 minutes more.

Nutritions

Per Serving: 120 calories; protein 3.9g; carbohydrates 12.2g; fat 7.5g; sodium 48.8mg.

Chilaquiles

Prep:

20 mins

Cook:

30 mins

Total:

50 mins

Servings:

8

Yield:

8 servings

Ingredients

1 tablespoon vegetable oil

1 ½ cups thinly sliced red onion

1 jalapeno pepper, seeded and minced

2 (16 ounce) jars salsa verde

1 pound shredded cooked skinless, boneless chicken breast

1 (10 ounce) bag tortilla chips

1 (2.25 ounce) can sliced black olives, drained

¼ cup chopped fresh cilantro

8 eggs

1 dash salt

1 dash ground black pepper

½ cup crumbled cotija cheese

4 radishes, sliced, or to taste

1 avocado, sliced, or to taste

Directions

1

Preheat the oven to 400 degrees F (200 degrees C).

2

Heat oil in a large skillet over medium heat. Add onion and jalapeno; cook, stirring occasionally, until onion begins to brown, about 10 minutes. Transfer to a very large bowl. Add salsa, chicken, chips, olives, and cilantro. Toss to coat, breaking chips slightly. Transfer to a 9x13-inch baking dish.

3

Use the bottom of a custard or measuring cup to make 8 indentations in the chip mixture. Crack 1 egg into each indentation. Sprinkle eggs evenly with salt and black pepper.

4

Bake until eggs are set and tortilla chips are softened and browned at edges, 20 to 25 minutes. Sprinkle with cotija cheese, radishes, and avocado.

Nutritions

Per Serving: 470 calories; protein 27g; carbohydrates 35.2g; fat 24.3g; cholesterol 237.2mg; sodium 838.7mg.

Cucumber Soup

Prep:

15 mins

Additional:

30 mins

Total:

45 mins

Servings:

4

Yield:

4 servings

Ingredients

4 cucumbers - peeled, quartered, and seeded
1 (14.5 ounce) can chicken broth
1 cup chopped tomato
¼ cup fresh lime juice
⅛ teaspoon cayenne pepper

Directions

1

Place 2 cucumbers in a blender; pour in chicken stock. Blend cucumber mixture until smooth and pureed; pour cucumber puree into a large bowl.

2

Chop the remaining 2 cucumbers. Stir chopped cucumbers, tomato, lime juice, and cayenne pepper into pureed cucumber until well mixed. Refrigerate until chilled, at least 30 minutes.

Nutritions

Per Serving: 43 calories; protein 2.1g; carbohydrates 8.6g; fat 0.7g; cholesterol 2.3mg; sodium 441.6mg.

CHAPTER 6: SNACKS AND SIDES RECIPES

Citrus Salad Sauce

Prep Time: 10 minutes
Cook Time: 0 minutes
Yield: About 3/4 cup 1x

INGREDIENTS

2 tablespoons orange juice, plus zest of 1/2 orange
1/2 cup olive oil
1/2 tablespoon Dijon mustard
1 tablespoon lemon juice
1/2 teaspoon maple syrup
Fresh ground black pepper
1/4 teaspoon kosher salt

DIRECTIONS

Zest the orange. In a medium bowl, mix the orange juice, orange zest, lemon juice, mustard, maple syrup, salt and a grind of fresh black pepper.
Gradually whisk in the olive oil 1 tablespoon at a time (8 tablespoons total), until creamy and emulsified. If desired, season with additional salt.

Golden Turmeric Sauce

PREP TIME5 MINS
COOK TIME20 MINS
Serves: 4 cups

INGREDIENTS

2 tbsp coconut oil
2-inch piece of ginger, peeled and minced
2 cloves garlic, minced
1 onion, roughly chopped
1 cup bone broth
2 tbsp turmeric powder
2 cups white sweet potato, cubed
¼ tsp cinnamon powder
1½ tsp sea salt
½ tsp ginger powder
1 can BPA-free coconut milk
1 lemon, juiced

DIRECTIONS

Heat the coconut oil in the bottom of a medium saucepan on medium heat. When the fat has melted and the pan is hot, add the onions and cook, stirring, for five minutes, or until lightly browned and translucent.

Add the garlic and fresh ginger and cook, stirring, for another minute, or until fragrant.

Add the bone broth, sweet potato, turmeric, ginger, cinnamon, and sea salt to the pot and mix. Bring to a boil and then cover and turn down to a simmer on low to cook for 10 minutes, or until sweet potatoes are just soft. When finished, turn off the heat and let the mixture cool for 5 minutes.

Place the coconut milk and lemon in the blender with the turmeric mixture, and (being careful to use a towel over the lid to protect your hands) blend until fully smooth and combined.

Your turmeric sauce is ready to be served as an accompaniment to protein, vegetables, stored, or used in another recipe!

Dijon Mustard Vinaigrette

Total Time: 5 minutes
Makes: about 1 cup

Ingredients

1/4 cup white wine vinegar (or lemon juice)
2 tablespoons Dijon mustard
1/2 cup olive oil
1 garlic clove, minced
1/4 teaspoon black pepper
1/2 teaspoon coarse salt

Directions

Combine ingredients in a bowl.
Whisk until smooth and everything has emulsified.
Adjust seasoning with salt & pepper, to taste.

Nutrition

Serving Size: 2 tablespoons
Calories: 113
Sugar: 0.1g
Sodium: 165g
Fat: 12.8g
Saturated Fat: 1.8g
Carbohydrates: 0.5g
Fiber: 0.2g
Protein: 0.2g
Cholesterol: 0

Chunky Tomato Sauce

PREP TIME5 mins
COOK TIME35 mins
TOTAL TIME40 mins

Ingredients

1 tbsp oil
3 cloves garlic finely diced
1/2 tsp salt
2 onions finely diced
2 stalks celery finely diced
6 cups chopped tomatoes
4 leaves fresh basil
1 carrot finely diced
1/4 tsp chili flakes
1 tsp dried oregano
1/2 tbsp red wine vinegar

DIRECTIONS

In a large pot on medium heat, heat the oil. Add in the onions and garlic, sprinkle with salt and cook for 4 minutes until the garlic becomes fragrant. Add in the diced celery and carrot and cook for another 5 minutes.

Add in the chopped tomatoes, basil, oregano, chilli flakes and red wine vinegar and leave everything to cook for 20 - 25 minutes.

Once the tomatoes are completely stewed and the sauce has thickened you can serve it as it or use an immersion blender (or transfer to a blender) and blend until completely smooth.

Yogurt Garlic Sauce

YIELDMakes about 1 cup

INGREDIENTS

1 teaspoon chopped garlic

1 cup plain yogurt (preferably whole-milk)

1 tablespoon fresh lemon juice

1/2 teaspoon kosher salt

PREPARATION

Mash garlic to a paste with salt using a mortar and pestle (or mince and mash with a heavy knife). Stir together garlic paste, yogurt, and lemon juice.

Cooks' note:

Sauce may be made 1 day ahead and chilled, covered.

Pumpkin Bites

Prep:15 mins
Additional:30 mins
Servings:6

Ingredients

½ cup almond flour

¼ cup almond butter

½ cup gluten-free rolled oats

¼ cup pumpkin puree

½ teaspoon almond extract

¼ teaspoon ground cloves

1 packet stevia sugar substitute (such as Truvia®)

¼ teaspoon ground nutmeg

1 pinch sea salt

½ teaspoon ground cinnamon

Directions

Combine oats, almond flour, almond butter, pumpkin puree, stevia sugar substitute, almond extract, cloves, nutmeg, cinnamon, and sea salt in a food processor; pulse just until combined.
Roll mixture into balls and arrange on a plate or baking sheet; refrigerate until set, at least 30 minutes.

Nutrition

158 calories; protein 4.8g; carbohydrates 10.2g; fat 11.8g; sodium 125.5mg.

Chimicurri Sauce

Prep: 10 min
Resting: 10 min
Total: 10 min

INGREDIENTS

1/2 cup olive oil
1/2 cup finely chopped parsley
3-4 cloves garlic , finely chopped or minced
2 tablespoons red wine vinegar
3/4 teaspoon dried oregano
1 level teaspoon coarse salt
pepper , to taste (about 1/2 teaspoon)
2 small red chilies , or 1 red chili, deseeded and finely chopped (about 1 tablespoon finely chopped chili)

DIRECTIONS

Mix all ingredients together in a bowl. Allow to sit for 5-10 minutes to release all of the flavours into the oil before using. Ideally, let it sit for more than 2 hours, if time allows.

Chimichurri can be prepared earlier than needed, and refrigerated for 24 hours, if needed.

Use to baste meats (chicken or steaks) while grilling or barbecuing. We don't use it as a marinade, but choose to baste our meats with chimichurri instead. However, you can use it as a marinade if you wish. Also, add a couple of tablespoons over your steak to serve.

NUTRITION

Calories: 128kcal | Carbohydrates: 1g | Fat: 13g | Saturated
Fat: 1g | Sodium: 3mg | Potassium: 61mg | Vitamin
A: 425IU | Vitamin C: 21.5mg | Calcium: 12mg | Iron: 0.5mg

Mini Zucchini Pizza Bites Mini Zucchini Pà

Pizza BitesPrep Time10 mins
Cook Time10 mins
Servings6 servings

Ingredients

2 large zucchini
1 teaspoon oregano
½ cup low carb pizza or tomato sauce
2 cups mozzarella cheese
pizza toppings as desired
¼ cup parmesan cheese

Directions

Preheat oven to 450°F. Line a baking pan with foil and set aside.
Slice Zucchini ¼" thick and arrange on prepared baking sheet.
Top zucchini slices with pizza sauce, oregano, cheese and your favorite
pizza toppings.
Bake 5 min or until zucchini is tender. Broil 5 min or until cheese is
bubbly and melted.

Nutrition

Calories: 145kcal | Carbohydrates: 4g | Protein: 10g | Fat: 9g | Satura
ted
Fat: 5g | Cholesterol: 32mg | Sodium: 413mg | Potassium: 266mg | F

iber: 1g | Sugar: 2g | Vitamin A: 505IU | Vitamin C: 13.1mg | Calcium: 256mg | Iron: 0.8mg

Chipotle Wings

Servings: 8

Ingredients

4 lb chicken wing and drumette(2 kg)
¼ cup cornstarch(30 g)
¼ cup lime juice(60 mL)
2 teaspoons salt, divided
1 ½ cups chipotle peppers in adobo(300 g)
1 teaspoon garlic powder
¼ cup honey(85 g)

Directions

Pat dry chicken and place in a large mixing bowl or plastic bag. Toss
with cornstarch, garlic powder, and one teaspoon of kosher salt.
Place chicken in a single layer on a cookie sheet or wire rack and
refrigerate for at least an hour, up to overnight.
In a food processor or blender, combine chipotles, lime juice, honey,
and the remaining salt. Puree until smooth. Set aside until ready to
grill.
Preheat grill to medium high heat. Grill wings until just starting to
brown on the underside, about 5 minutes, then flip and repeat.
Using a basting brush, coat the top side of the wings with chipotle
puree. Flip and cook until exterior just starts to char. Baste the other
side, flip and repeat.
Remove wings from heat and let cool for at least 5 minutes. Serve with
your preferred garnish and dipping sauce.

Nutritions

Calories 518

Fat 35g
Carbs 17g
Fiber 0g
Sugar 12g
Protein 34g

Green Tomatillo Salsa

PREP TIME10 mins
COOK TIME15 mins
YIELDS3 cups

Ingredients

1 1/2 lb tomatillos
2 cloves garlic
1/2 cup cilantro leaves
1/2 cup chopped white onion
2 Jalapeño peppers OR 2 serrano peppers, stemmed, seeded and
chopped
1 Tbsp fresh lime juice
Salt to taste

Directions

Remove papery husks from tomatillos and rinse well
3 ways to cook the tomatillos
2a Oven Roasting Method
Cut the tomatillos in half and place cut side down on a foil-lined
baking sheet. Add a few garlic cloves in their skin (if using) Place
under a broiler for about 6-8 minutes to lightly blacken the skins of the
tomatillos.
2b Pan Roasting Method
Coat the bottom of a skillet with a little vegetable oil. Heat on high
heat. Place the tomatillos in the pan and sear on one side, then flip
over and brown on the other side. Remove from heat.
2c Boiling Method
Place tomatillos in a saucepan, cover with water. Bring to a boil and
simmer for 5 minutes. Remove tomatillos with a slotted spoon.
Pulse in blender

219

Place the cooked tomatillos, lime juice, onions, garlic (if using), cilantro, chili peppers in a blender or food processor and pulse until all ingredients are finely chopped and mixed.

Season to taste with salt.

Cool in refrigerator.

Serve with chips or as a salsa accompaniment to Mexican dishes.

Citrus Relish

Servings 1

Ingredients

1½ pink grapefruits
1½ navel oranges
3 lemons
3 tablespoons sugar
1 tablespoon olive oil
1 teaspoon kosher salt
¼ cup fresh parsley leaves
Flaky sea salt (such as Maldon)

Directions

Preheat oven to 350°. Slice ½ grapefruit, ½ orange, and 1 lemon crosswise into paper-thin rounds; remove seeds. Toss in a medium bowl with sugar, oil, and kosher salt. Roast on a parchment-lined baking sheet until golden in spots and crisp, 20–30 minutes; let cool. Meanwhile, cut all peel and white pith from remaining grapefruit, orange, and lemons. Working over a medium bowl, cut along sides of membranes to release segments into bowl; discard membranes. Tear roasted citrus into pieces and toss with segments, breaking up larger segments. Stir in parsley; season with sea salt.
DO AHEAD: Citrus can be roasted and segmented 1 day ahead. Store roasted citrus wrapped tightly at room temperature; cover and chill citrus segments.

Pita Wedges

YIELDS:12 servings
PREP TIME:0 hours 3 mins
COOK TIME:0 hours 15 mins

Ingredients

6 pieces Pita Bread
1/2 c. Olive Oil
3 tbsp. Kosher Salt

Directions

Preheat the oven to 375 F.

Cut the pita pieces into six wedges each. Lay the wedges on a foil-lined baking sheet and brush both sides generously with olive oil. Sprinkle both sides with salt, then bake them for 15 to 18 minutes until they're golden brown and crisp.

Serve warm or at room temperature with whatever dip you want!

Grilled Vegetables

Prep Time 30 minutes
Servings 4

Ingredients

2 portabello mushrooms
1 eggplant
1 yellow squash
1 zucchini
1 bunch thick asparagus
1 red bell pepper
1 onion
2 tablespoons extra virgin olive oil
1 tablespoon freshly ground black pepper
1 tablespoon kosher salt

Directions

Prepare the grill with clean grates and preheat to medium heat, 350°F to 450°F.

Trim the ends of the eggplant, zucchini, yellow squash and onion and cut into 1/3" to 1/2" slices. Seed the red bell pepper and cut into quarters. Trim the ends of the asparagus.

Drizzle the vegetables with olive oil and sprinkle evenly with salt and pepper. Grill the vegetables with the lid closed until tender and lightly charred all over, about 8 to 10 minutes for the bell peppers, onion, and mushroom; 5-7 minutes for the yellow squash, zucchini, and eggplant and asparagus.

Serve warm or at room temperature.

Nutrition

Fat 8g12%

223

Saturated Fat 1g6%
Sodium 1760mg77%
Potassium 1021mg29%
Carbohydrates 21g7%
Fiber 9g38%
Sugar 12g13%
Protein 6g

Dilled Carrots

Prep:10 mins
Cook:10 mins
Servings:4

Ingredients

3 cups peeled and sliced carrots
2 tablespoons brown sugar
1 ½ tablespoons chopped fresh dill
 tablespoons butter
½ teaspoon black pepper
½ teaspoon salt

Directions

Place carrots in a skillet and pour in just enough water to cover. Bring to a boil over medium heat; simmer until water has evaporated and the carrots are tender. Stir in butter, brown sugar, dill, salt, and pepper.

Nutrition

117 calories; protein 1g; carbohydrates 16.1g; fat 6g; cholesterol 15.3mg; sodium 400.7mg.

Fajita Flavor Marinade

Prep:20 mins
Cook:10 mins
Additional:2 hrs
Servings:4

Ingredients

1 pound beef round steak, cut into thin strips
1 yellow bell pepper, cut into thin strips
1 red onion, thinly sliced
2 anaheim chile peppers, thinly sliced
1 red bell pepper, cut into thin strips
6 tablespoons olive oil
4 large cloves garlic, crushed
1 (1.27 ounce) packet spicy fajita seasoning

Directions

Combine beef strips, red bell pepper, yellow bell pepper, onion, anaheim chile peppers, fajita seasoning, olive oil, and garlic in a large bowl. Cover and refrigerate for at least 2 hours.
Heat a large skillet over medium heat; cook and stir the beef and vegetable mixture in hot skillet until beef is no longer pink in the center and vegetables are tender, about 10 minutes.

Nutrition

366 calories; protein 22.9g; carbohydrates 16.4g; fat 23.8g; cholesterol 56.3mg; sodium 659.5mg.

Quick Pesto

Prep: 20 mins
Total:20 mins
Servings:24

Ingredients

1 ½ cups baby spinach leaves
½ cup toasted pine nuts
½ cup grated Parmesan cheese
¾ cup fresh basil leaves
¾ teaspoon kosher salt
½ teaspoon freshly ground black pepper
1 tablespoon fresh lemon juice
4 cloves garlic, peeled and quartered
½ cup extra-virgin olive oil
½ teaspoon lemon zest

Directions

Blend the spinach, basil, pine nuts, Parmesan cheese, garlic, salt, pepper, lemon juice, lemon zest, and 2 tablespoons olive oil in a food processor until nearly smooth, scraping the sides of the bowl with a spatula as necessary. Drizzle the remaining olive oil into the mixture while processing until smooth.

Nutrition

67 calories; protein 1.5g; carbohydrates 0.8g; fat 6.6g; cholesterol 1.5mg; sodium 87.2mg

Rutabaga Latkes

Prep Time10 mins
Cook Time20 mins
Servings: 10 Latkes

Ingredients

1 lb. peeled, grated rutabaga (approx. 3 cups)
1 egg, lightly beaten
1 Tbsp. coconut flour
1 scallion, minced
3-4 Tbsp. raw, shelled hemp seeds
1 tsp. salt
A few gratings of fresh nutmeg
Pepper to taste
Olive oil for frying

Directions

In a large bowl, add grated rutabaga, minced scallion, beaten egg, coconut flour, hemp seeds, salt, pepper and nutmeg. Mix well.
In a large skillet, heat a good tablespoon of olive oil between medium low and medium heat. Working in batches of 3 latkes, spoon about 2 tablespoons of mixture per latke into skillet, spreading into 3 to 4 inch rounds and frying until the edges begin to brown. Flip and fry until other side is golden brown. Repeat with remaining latke mixture, adding another good tablespoon of olive oil to the skillet for each batch.
When latkes are done frying, place in warm oven on wire racks on a rimmed baking sheet. This keeps latkes crispy until ready to serve.

Crack Slaw

Prep Time10 minutes
Cook Time:25 minutes
Servings4

Ingredients

1 pound lean ground beef or chicken or turkey

2 tablespoons sesame seed oil

6-7 cups coleslaw mix

4 cloves garlic minced

2 tablespoons soy sauce

2 teaspoons white vinegar

1-2 tablespoons sriracha

1/2 teaspoon white sugar OR splenda for low carb

1/2 teaspoon pepper

1 teaspoon toasted sesame seeds

1/2 teaspoon salt

2-3 tablespoons green onion chopped

Directions

In a large skillet, fry the ground beef until cooked and no longer pink. Drain and return to the stove.

Push the ground beef to the side and add the sesame seed oil in the space. Add in the garlic and fry for 2-3 minutes, then mix into the ground beef.

Add in the coleslaw mix. Drizzle with sriracha, vinegar, soy sauce and sprinkle with the sugar, salt and pepper. Fry for another 5 minutes until the cabbage is wilted to your liking.

Plate, then sprinkle with the toasted sesame seed and green onions.

Nutrition

Calories: 255kcal, Carbohydrates: 8g, Protein: 26g, Fat: 12g, Saturated Fat: 3g, Cholesterol: 70mg, Sodium: 974mg, Potassium: 601mg, Fiber: 2g, Sugar: 3g, Vitamin A: 135IU, Vitamin C: 42.3mg, Calcium: 58mg, Iron: 3.5mg

Addictive Pretzels

Servings: 10
Cook: 1 hour
Prep: 30 mins

Ingredients

32 ounces bag unsalted pretzels
3 teaspoons dried dill weed
2 tablespoons Hidden Valley® Ranch Salad Dressing and Seasoning mix
3 teaspoons garlic powder
1 cup canola oil

Directions

Preheat oven to 175° F.
Spread the pretzels out on two 18" x 13" cookie sheets, so that pretzels lay flat. Use whole bite-size pretzels or break large-size pretzels into pieces.
Mix the garlic powder and dill together. Set aside half of the seasonings. To the other half, add the dry salad dressing mix and 3/4 cup canola oil. Pour evenly over the pretzels and use your hands to make sure pretzels are evenly coated.
Bake for 1 hour, flipping the pretzels every 15 minutes.
Remove the pretzels from the oven. Let the pretzels cool, then toss with remaining garlic powder, dill weed and oil. Enjoy!

Nutrition

Calories 184
Protein 2 g
Carbohydrates 22 g

Fat 8 g
Cholesterol 0 mg
Sodium 60 mg
Potassium 43 mg
Phosphorus 28 mg
Calcium 2 mg
Fiber 1.0 g

Turnip Chips

Prep Time10 mins
Cook Time25 mins
Servings4

INGREDIENTS

2 large turnips skin peeled
½ teaspoon salt
3 tablespoons olive oil
¼ teaspoon pepper

DIRECTIONS

Pre-heat oven to 400 degrees and line two baking sheets with tin foil. Spray foil with non-stick cooking spray.

Using a mandoline, thinly slice the turnips into chips and place in a large mixing bowl.

Drizzle turnip slices with olive oil, salt and pepper. Toss well to coat evenly.

Spread chips in an even layer on baking sheets. Be careful not to over-crowd.

Bake for 20-25 minutes, turning once halfway through to ensure even cooking.

Let cool 10 minutes to continue crisping then serve.

NUTRITION

Calories: 115kcalCarbohydrates: 5.9gProtein: 0.8gFat: 10.2gSaturated Fat: 1.4gPolyunsaturated Fat: 8.8gTrans Fat: 0gCholesterol: 0mgSodium: 352mgFiber: 1.6gSugar: 3.5g

Cashew Sour Cream

Prep:

5 mins

Additional:

8 hrs

Total:

8 hrs 5 mins

Servings:

10

Yield:

1 1/4 cups

Ingredients

1 cup raw cashews

7 tablespoons water

2 teaspoons fresh lemon juice

2 teaspoons rice vinegar

½ teaspoon kosher salt

Directions

1

Place cashews in a bowl and cover with a few inches of water. Let soak until soft, 8 hours to overnight.

2

Drain and rinse cashews; transfer to a high-powered blender. Add 4 tablespoons water, lemon juice, vinegar, and salt. Blend until cashews are finely ground. Scrape down the sides of the blender and add remaining water; blend until very smooth.

3

Transfer cashew cream to a jar with a tight-fitting lid and store in the refrigerator.

Nutritions

Per Serving: 76 calories; protein 2.5g; carbohydrates 4.2g; fat 6g; sodium 98mg.

Cucumber Yogurt

Prep:

20 mins

Total:

20 mins

Servings:

4

Yield:

4 servings

Ingredients

4 small seedless cucumbers - peeled and grated

1 tablespoon fresh lemon juice

1 bunch fresh mint leaves, chopped

1 bunch fresh dill, chopped

2 cloves garlic, crushed

2 cups plain yogurt

1 tablespoon olive oil

1 teaspoon salt (Optional)

¼ cup raisins (Optional)

Directions

1

Combine the grated cucumber, lemon juice, mint, dill, garlic, yogurt, olive oil, and salt in a large mixing bowl; stir with a large spoon. Pour the mixture into a blender; blend on high speed until smooth. Serve immediately or chill in refrigerator until ready to serve. Divide the soup between four bowls; top each serving with about 1 tablespoon raisins.

Nutritions

Per Serving: 168 calories; protein 8.5g; carbohydrates 22.9g; fat 5.8g; cholesterol 7.4mg; sodium 676.6mg.

Mango Chiller

Prep:

15 mins

Cook:

45 mins

Total:

1 hr

Servings:

24

Yield:

3 cups

Ingredients

2 pounds ripe mangoes
1 ½ cups white sugar
¾ cup water
3 saffron threads (Optional)

Directions

1

Boil, steam, or microwave the whole mangoes until soft. Cool, then remove the peel and inner seed; place the mango pulp in a large bowl. Use a fork or potato masher to mash the pulp well.

2

Place the sugar and water in a large saucepan over low heat, stir mixture, and bring to a boil. When mixture begins boiling, increase heat to medium-high. Continue boiling until fine, soft threads form, 270 degrees F (135 degrees C). Stir in the mango pulp, add the saffron threads, if desired, and boil until the mixture thickens, about 5 minutes.

3

Pour cooked jam into sterilized jars and seal according to canning directions.

Nutritions

Per Serving: 73 calories; protein 0.2g; carbohydrates 18.9g; fat 0.1g; sodium 1mg.

Roasted Radishes

Prep:

15 mins

Cook:

15 mins

Total:

30 mins

Servings:

4

Yield:

4 servings

Ingredients

2 bunches radishes, trimmed

2 tablespoons extra-virgin olive oil

1 teaspoon ground thyme

salt to taste

½ lemon, juiced

Directions

1

Preheat oven to 450 degrees F (230 degrees C). Line a baking sheet with aluminum foil.

2

Cut radishes into halves; cut any large radishes into quarters. Stir olive oil and thyme together in a bowl and toss radishes in mixture to coat. Spread radishes onto prepared baking sheet; sprinkle with salt.

3

Roast in the preheated oven until tender but firm in the centers, tossing every 5 minutes, 15 to 20 minutes. Drizzle with lemon juice.

Nutritions

Per Serving: 70 calories; protein 0.3g; carbohydrates 2.1g; fat 6.8g; sodium 16.6mg.

Cottage Cheese

Prep:

10 mins

Cook:

10 mins

Total:

20 mins

Servings:

1

Yield:

1 breakfast bowl

Ingredients

2 slices bacon, chopped

2 medium fresh mushrooms, chopped

1 tablespoon minced green onions (including green tops)

salt and ground black pepper to taste

2 eggs, lightly beaten

½ cup cottage cheese

Directions

1

Cook bacon in a small nonstick skillet over medium heat until browned, 4 to 5 minutes. Transfer bacon to a paper towel-lined bowl, reserving bacon grease in a small bowl.

2

Return skillet to medium-high heat and add 1 teaspoon reserved bacon grease. Cook mushrooms and green onions until lightly browned, 3 to

4 minutes. Season with salt and pepper. Transfer to a small bowl and keep warm.

3

Return skillet to medium-high heat and add 1 teaspoon reserved bacon grease. Add eggs and scramble until cooked through, 2 to 3 minutes. Season with salt and pepper. Remove from heat and keep warm.

4

Place cottage cheese into a microwave-safe bowl. Heat on 50% power for 60 to 90 seconds, or until warm, stirring halfway through. Drain any liquid that has been released and transfer cottage cheese into one side of a single-serving bowl. Place scrambled eggs into the other side of the bowl. Top with mushroom mixture and bacon. Serve immediately.

Nutritions

Per Serving: 366 calories; protein 34.5g; carbohydrates 5.7g; fat 22.7g; cholesterol 408.7mg; sodium 1169.3mg.

Garlic Oyster Crackers

Prep:

10 mins

Cook:

20 mins

Total:

30 mins

Servings:

24

Yield:

24 servings

Ingredients

¾ cup vegetable oil

1 (1 ounce) package dry Ranch-style dressing mix

½ teaspoon dried dill weed

¼ teaspoon lemon pepper

¼ teaspoon garlic powder

1 (12 ounce) package oyster crackers

Directions

1

Preheat oven to 275 degrees F (135 degrees C).

2

In a mixing bowl, whisk together vegetable oil, ranch-style dressing mix, dill weed, lemon pepper and garlic powder. Pour this spice mixture over the crackers in a medium bowl, and stir until the crackers are coated. Arrange the crackers on a large baking sheet.

3

Bake in the preheated 275 degrees F (135 degrees C) oven for 15 to 20 minutes.

Nutritions

Per Serving: 128 calories; protein 1.1g; carbohydrates 9.7g; fat 9.4g; sodium 354.3mg.

CHAPTER 7: DESSERTS

Pear Sorbet

SERVES 6
COOKS IN25 MINUTES PLUS FREEZING TIME

NUTRITION

Calories21311%
Fat0.2g0%
Saturates0.0g0%
Sugars49.8g55%
Protein0.7g1%
Carbs49.8g19%

Ingredients

200 g caster sugar
1 kg soft pears , peeled, quartered and cores removed
55 ml grappa , or to taste
1 lemon , juice and zest of
200 ml water

Directions

Sorbets are always a nice way to finish a meal if you don't want
anything too heavy. They can also be used as palate cleansers between
courses. Either way, a sorbet is pretty much always made the same way
– a fruit purée is mixed with a little stock syrup in the right quantity to
make it freeze. It will become really shiny and soft to scoop.
This particular recipe for pear and grappa sorbet is a wicked combo
and one of my favourites, so give it a bash. It's great served in a bowl

with lovely soft fruits scattered over the top. A good-quality vodka instead of grappa would be quite interesting and, without wanting to sound like a nutcase, absinthe would be nice too, but to be honest most good supermarkets and off-licences sell grappa these days. Nardini is a particularly good brand.

This recipe will make enough for 6 people to have a couple of scoops each, but for 4 you can make this amount and keep the rest in the freezer for another day. I suggest you use a fairly shallow earthenware or thick porcelain dish that you can put in the freezer beforehand – this speeds up the freezing process for the sorbet.

Try to get really ripe pears – even the ones they sell cheaply in the market. If they're really really ripe and soft to the touch, simply remove the skin and put the flesh into a bowl – you won't need to cook them at all. This is how I did it in Italy when the fruit guy called Pippo at the weekly Terranuova Bracciolini market near Montevarchi gave me a whole tray of pears for free. Go and say hello and he might do the same for you!

First of all put the sugar and water into a pan on the hob. Bring to the boil, then reduce the heat and simmer for 3 minutes. Add your quartered pears and, unless they're super soft, continue to simmer for 5 minutes. Remove from the heat, leave to one side for 5 minutes, then add the lemon juice (minus the pips) and zest. Pour everything into a food processor and whiz to a purée, then push the mixture through a coarse sieve into the dish in which you want to serve it. Add the grappa, give it a good stir, and taste. The grappa shouldn't be overbearing or too powerful – it should be subtle and should work well with the pears. However, different brands do vary in strength and flavour, so add to taste. (This isn't an excuse to add the whole bottle, though, because if you use too much alcohol the sorbet won't freeze.) Put the dish into the freezer and whisk it up with a fork every half-hour – you'll see it becoming pale in colour. After a couple of hours it will be ready. The texture should be nice and scoopable. Delicious served with ventagli or other delicate crunchy biscuits.

Chocolate Sorbet

Prep:5 mins
Cook:10 mins
Additional:3 hrs 20 mins
Servings:4

Ingredients

1 cup white sugar
⅛ teaspoon sea salt
2 cups water
2 tablespoons brewed espresso or strong coffee
½ teaspoon almond extract
⅔ cup unsweetened cocoa powder

Directions

Mix sugar, cocoa powder, and sea salt in a large saucepan. Stir in water, espresso, and almond extract. Bring to a boil over medium heat. Once the sugar has dissolved and mixture is smooth, remove from heat and stir in the coffee liqueur. Transfer mixture to a bowl, cover, and chill completely in the refrigerator or using an ice bath.
Pour mixture into an ice cream maker and churn until slightly thickened according to manufacturer's Directions, about 20 minutes. Transfer mixture to an airtight container and freeze until firm enough to scoop, 3 to 4 hours or overnight.

Nutrition

255 calories; protein 2.8g; carbohydrates 60.6g; fat 2g; sodium 63.3mg.

Blueberry Sorbet

Prep:5 mins
Additional:6 hrs
Servings:10

Ingredients

3 cups fresh pink grapefruit juice
1 ½ cups white sugar, or to taste
3 cups fresh or frozen blueberries

Directions

Pour the grapefruit juice, blueberries, sugar, and vodka into a blender, and blend until the sugar is dissolved and the mixture is smooth, 2 to 4 minutes.
Pour the mixture into a container, and freeze until solid, 3 to 4 hours. Thoroughly stir the sorbet to break up the ice crystals to a slushy consistency, and return to freezer until firm, about 3 hours. Store in the freezer in a covered container.

Nutrition

197 calories; protein 0.7g; carbohydrates 43.1g; fat 0.2g; sodium 1.3mg.

Zesty Mousse

Ingredients

1 package (7g) Unflavoured gelatin
2/3 cup Plain yogurt
1 tbsp Grated lemon rind
½ cup Lemon juice
1 cup Granulated sugar
1 cup Whipping cream
¼ cup Cold water

Directions

In saucepan, sprinkle gelatin over cold water; let stand for 1 minute to soften.
Stir over low heat until gelatin dissolves.
Stir in lemon rind, lemon juice and half of the sugar.
Stir in yogurt.
In bowl, whip cream with remaining sugar; fold into lemon mixture.
Spoon into parfait glasses or serving dish.
Cover and refrigerate for 2 hours.

Makes 6-8 servings.

Cinnamon Lemon Tea

Ingredients

8 cups filtered water
1 fresh ginger root, peeled and sliced
1 bunch mint leaves
8 cinnamon sticks
2 lemon wedge, quartered

Directions

Fill pot with filtered water.
Add lemon wedges, mint leaves, cinnamon sticks and ginger.
Bring water to a boil.
Reduce stove to simmer and enjoy throughout the day or remove from stove and pour into a glass jar to drink throughout the week. Can store in refrigerator.

Chia Chocolate Pudding

Prep:15 mins
Additional:8 hrs 15 mins
Servings:2

Ingredients

1 cup milk
1 tablespoon chocolate covered hemp seeds, or to taste
2 tablespoons cocoa powder
1 tablespoon brown sugar
1 tablespoon white sugar
¼ cup chia seeds
¼ teaspoon vanilla extract
1 tiny pinch salt
½ teaspoon instant coffee granules

Directions

Whisk milk, chia seeds, cocoa powder, brown sugar, white sugar, coffee granules, vanilla extract, and salt together in a bowl until pudding is smooth. Let sit for 5 minutes; stir. Repeat sitting and stirring process at least 2 times.
Cover the bowl with plastic wrap and refrigerate, 8 hours to overnight. Spoon into bowls and top with chocolate hemp seeds.

Nutrition

239 calories; protein 8.1g; carbohydrates 32.6g; fat 10g; cholesterol 9.8mg; sodium 152.8mg.

Almond Cookie

Prep:40 mins
Cook:15 mins
Servings:48
Prep:

Ingredients

2 ¾ cups sifted all-purpose flour
1 teaspoon almond extract
 cup white sugar
½ teaspoon salt
1 cup lard
1 egg
½ teaspoon baking soda
48 almonds

Directions

Preheat oven to 325 degrees F .
Sift flour, sugar, baking soda and salt together into a bowl. Cut in the lard until mixture resembles cornmeal. Add egg and almond extract. Mix well.
Roll dough into 1-inch balls. Set them 2 inches apart on an ungreased cookie sheet. Place an almond on top of each cookie and press down to flatten slightly.
Bake in the preheated oven until the edges of the cookies are golden brown, 16 to 18 minutes.

Nutrition

89 calories; protein 1.1g; carbohydrates 9.9g; fat 5.1g; cholesterol 7.9mg; sodium 38.9mg.

Apple Chia Pudding

Active:10 mins
Total:8 hrs 10 mins
Servings:1

Ingredients

½ cup unsweetened almond milk or other nondairy milk

2 tablespoons chia seeds

¼ teaspoon vanilla extract

1 tablespoon chopped toasted pecans, divided

¼ teaspoon ground cinnamon

½ cup diced apple, divided

2 teaspoons pure maple syrup

Directions

Stir almond milk (or other nondairy milk), chia, maple syrup, vanilla and cinnamon together in a small bowl. Cover and refrigerate for at least 8 hours and up to 3 days.

When ready to serve, stir well. Spoon about half the pudding into a serving glass (or bowl) and top with half the apple and pecans. Add the rest of the pudding and top with the remaining apple and pecans.

Nutrition

233 calories; protein 4.8g; carbohydrates 27.7g; dietary fiber 10.1g; sugars 14.4g; fat 12.7g; saturated fat 1.1g; vitamin a iu 297.7IU; vitamin c 3mg; folate 13.5mcg; calcium 385.9mg; iron 2.1mg; magnesium 84.7mg; potassium 224.2mg; sodium 90.7mg; thiamin 0.2mg; added sugar 8g.

Banana Muffins

Prep:15 mins
Cook:30 mins

Servings:12

Ingredients

3 cups all-purpose flour
½ cup brown sugar
2 teaspoons ground cinnamon
1 cup white sugar
1 teaspoon baking soda
1 teaspoon ground nutmeg
1 teaspoon salt
2 teaspoons baking powder
2 cups mashed ripe bananas
1 cup coconut milk
1 cup canola oil

Directions

Preheat oven to 350 degrees F. Grease 12 muffin cups or line with paper liners.
Mix flour, white sugar, brown sugar, cinnamon, baking powder, baking soda, nutmeg, and salt together in a large bowl. Stir bananas, canola oil, and coconut milk together in a separate bowl; mix banana mixture into flour mixture until just combined. Fill muffin cups with batter. Bake in the preheated oven until a tooth pick inserted in the center of a muffin comes out clean, 30 to 35 minutes.

Nutrition

451 calorics; protcin 4.1g; carbohydrates 59.2g; fat 23.2g; sodium 386mg.

Chocolaty Avocado Mousse

INGREDIENTS

2 large ripe avocados, peeled and stoned
3–4 tbsp runny honey, to taste
50g raw cacao powder
1 tsp vanilla extract

DIRECTIONS

Put the avocados into a food processor and blend until smooth.
Add 3 tablespoons of the honey with the vanilla and cacao powder
and blend again until completely combined. Taste and add more honey
if necessary.
Spoon the mousse into 8 shot or sweet wine glasses and put them into
the fridge for an hour before serving.

Pumpkin Cookies

Prep:20 mins
Cook:20 mins
Additional:40 mins
Servings:36

Ingredients

2 ½ cups all-purpose flour
1 teaspoon baking powder
2 teaspoons ground cinnamon
½ teaspoon ground nutmeg
1 teaspoon baking soda
½ teaspoon salt
½ cup butter, softened
1 ½ cups white sugar
½ teaspoon ground cloves
1 egg
1 teaspoon vanilla extract
2 cups confectioners' sugar
1 teaspoon vanilla extract
3 tablespoons milk
1 tablespoon melted butter
1 cup canned pumpkin puree

Directions

Preheat oven to 350 degrees F. Combine flour, baking powder, baking soda, cinnamon, nutmeg, ground cloves, and salt; set aside.
In a medium bowl, cream together the 1/2 cup of butter and white sugar. Add pumpkin, egg, and 1 teaspoon vanilla to butter mixture, and beat until creamy. Mix in dry ingredients. Drop on cookie sheet by tablespoonfuls; flatten slightly.

Bake for 15 to 20 minutes in the preheated oven. Cool cookies, then drizzle glaze with fork.

To Make Glaze: Combine confectioners' sugar, milk, 1 tablespoon melted butter, and 1 teaspoon vanilla. Add milk as needed, to achieve drizzling consistency.

Nutrition

122 calories; protein 1.2g; carbohydrates 22.4g; fat 3.2g; cholesterol 12.9mg; sodium 120.5mg.

Pumpkin Bread

Prep:15 mins
Cook:50 mins
Servings:24

Ingredients

1 (15 ounce) can pumpkin puree
4 eggs
⅔ cup water
3 cups white sugar
½ teaspoon ground cloves
3 ½ cups all-purpose flour
1 cup vegetable oil
2 teaspoons baking soda
1 teaspoon ground cinnamon
1 teaspoon ground nutmeg
1 ½ teaspoons salt
¼ teaspoon ground ginger

Directions

Preheat oven to 350 degrees F . Grease and flour three 7x3 inch loaf
pans.
In a large bowl, mix together pumpkin puree, eggs, oil, water and sugar
until well blended. In a separate bowl, whisk together the flour, baking
soda, salt, cinnamon, nutmeg, cloves and ginger. Stir the dry
ingredients into the pumpkin mixture until just blended. Pour into the
prepared pans.Bake for about 50 minutes in the preheated oven.
Loaves are done when toothpick inserted in center comes out clean.

Nutrition

263 calories; protein 3.1g; carbohydrates 40.6g; fat 10.3g; cholesterol 31mg; sodium 305.4mg.

Dutch Apple Pancake

Prep:15 mins
Cook:20 mins
Additional:10 mins
Servings:4

Ingredients

4 eggs
½ cup unbleached all-purpose flour
1 tablespoon sugar
1 pinch salt
½ teaspoon ground nutmeg
1 cup milk
½ teaspoon baking powder
1 teaspoon vanilla extract
½ teaspoon ground nutmeg
¼ cup unsalted butter
2 tablespoons unsalted butter, melted
½ cup white sugar, divided
½ teaspoon ground cinnamon
1 large tart apple - peeled, cored and sliced

Directions

In a large bowl, blend eggs, flour, baking powder, sugar and salt.
Gradually mix in milk, stirring constantly. Add vanilla, melted butter
and 1/2 teaspoon nutmeg. Let batter stand for 30 minutes or
overnight.
Preheat oven to 425 degrees F .
Melt butter in a 10 inch oven proof skillet, brushing butter up on the
sides of the pan. In a small bowl, combine 1/4 cup sugar, cinnamon
and 1/2 teaspoon nutmeg. Sprinkle mixture over the butter. Line the

263

pan with apple slices. Sprinkle remaining sugar over apples. Place pan over medium-high heat until the mixture bubbles, then gently pour the batter mixture over the apples.

Bake in preheated oven for 15 minutes. Reduce heat to 375 degrees F and bake for 10-12 minutes. Slide pancake onto serving platter and cut into wedges.

Nutrition

456 calories; protein 10.3g; carbohydrates 51.5g; fat 24g; cholesterol 236.6mg; sodium 182.2mg.

Vegan Pumpkin Ice Cream

Prep:10 mins
Cook:10 mins
Additional:3 hrs 30 mins
Servings:4

Ingredients

¼ cup soy creamer
2 tablespoons arrowroot powder
1 ¾ cups soy creamer
¾ cup brown sugar
1 cup pumpkin puree
1 cup soy milk
1 ½ teaspoons pumpkin pie spice
1 teaspoon vanilla extract

Directions

Mix 1/4 cup soy creamer with arrowroot and set aside. Whisk together
1 3/4 cup soy creamer, soy milk, brown sugar, pumpkin puree, vanilla
extract, and pumpkin pie spice in a saucepan over medium heat,
stirring frequently, until just boiling. Remove the pan from the heat;
stir in the arrowroot mixture to thicken. Set aside to cool for 30
minutes.
Fill cylinder of ice cream freezer; freeze according to manufacturer's
directions.

Nutrition

351 calories; protein 2.8g; carbohydrates 61.3g; fat 9.5g; sodium
231.2mg.

Sugar Cookies

Servings:24

Ingredients

1 ¼ cups white sugar
½ teaspoon cream of tartar
1 cup butter
3 egg yolks
2 ½ cups all-purpose flour
1 teaspoon baking soda
1 teaspoon vanilla extract

Directions

Preheat oven to 350 degrees F. Lightly grease 2 cookie sheets.
Cream together sugar and butter. Beat in egg yolks and vanilla.
Add flour, baking soda, and cream of tartar. Stir.
Form dough into walnut size balls and place 2 inches apart on cookie
sheet. Don't flatten. Bake 10 to 11 minutes, until tops are cracked and
just turning color.

Nutrition

163 calories; protein 1.8g; carbohydrates 20.5g; fat 8.4g; cholesterol
45.9mg; sodium 108.2mg

No-Bake Strawberry Cheesecake

Prep:30 mins
Additional:3 hrs 30 mins
Servings:10

Ingredients

1 (3 ounce) package strawberry-flavored gelatin (such as Jell-O®)
1 cup boiling water
1 cup white sugar
1 (5 ounce) can cold evaporated milk
1 teaspoon vanilla extract
1 (8 ounce) package cream cheese, softened
1 (9 inch) prepared graham cracker crust

Directions

Dissolve strawberry gelatin in boiling water in a bowl; cool in
refrigerator until thick, but not set, about 20 minutes.
Beat cream cheese, sugar, and vanilla extract together in a bowl until
smooth.
Beat evaporated milk in a separate bowl with an electric mixer until
whipped and thick. Gradually pour strawberry gelatin mixture into
evaporated milk, beating constantly. Fold cream cheese mixture into
gelatin-milk mixture to form cheesecake filling.
Set graham cracker crust on a baking sheet or plate to maintain
stability. Pour cheesecake filling into crust. Refrigerate until cake is set,
at least 3 1/2 hours.

Nutrition

324 calories; protein 4.4g; carbohydrates 44.9g; fat 14.8g; cholesterol
28.7mg; sodium 252.7mg.

Asian Pear Tort

Ingredients

2 cups (4 sticks) butter, ice cold and cut into ½-inch pieces
¼ cup heavy whipping cream
4 ¾ cups flour
3 egg yolks
2 cups powdered sugar

Directions

Beat butter and powdered sugar on medium speed in electric mixer
fitted with paddle attachment 5 minutes. Scrape down sides of bowl.
Add yolks 1 at a time with mixer on low speed. Add cream and mix at
medium speed 1 minute. Turn off mixer and add flour. Mix on low
speed until combined. Do not over mix.
Divide dough in half, wrap in plastic wrap and refrigerate 1 hour.

Brown sugar filling

Ingredients

1 ½ cups light brown sugar, packed
⅓ cup flour
¼ teaspoon cinnamon

Directions

Combine brown sugar, flour and cinnamon in bowl and stir until there are no lumps. Set aside.
Assembly

Asian Pear Crisp

Prep:15 mins
Cook:20 mins
Servings:2

Ingredients

2 pears - peeled, cored, and diced
¾ teaspoon ground cinnamon, divided
2 tablespoons quick-cooking oats
1 tablespoon all-purpose flour
1 teaspoon lemon juice
1 tablespoon salted butter, softened
1 tablespoon brown sugar

Directions

Preheat the air fryer to 360 degrees F .
Combine pears, lemon juice, and 1/4 teaspoon cinnamon in a medium
bowl. Toss to coat, then divide the mixture between 2 ramekins.
Combine oats, flour, brown sugar, and remaining 1/2 teaspoon
cinnamon in a small bowl. Mix in softened butter using a fork until
mixture is crumbly. Sprinkle over the pears.
Place the ramekins in the air fryer basket and cook until the pears are
soft and bubbling, 18 to 22 minutes.

Nutrition

234 calories; protein 2g; carbohydrates 46.3g; fat 6.4g; cholesterol
15.3mg; sodium 45.4mg.

Pie Crust

Prep:10 mins
Servings:8

Ingredients

1 ½ cups all-purpose flour
½ teaspoon salt
½ cup cold water
½ cup vegetable shortening

Directions

Mix shortening, flour, and salt together with a fork or a pastry blender until very crumbly. Add as much water as needed to hold together, and mix lightly with a fork.
Roll gently on a floured pastry cloth to about an inch larger than pie plate. Fold carefully in half, lift to pie plate, and unfold. Press into pan. For a single-crust pie, trim with a small knife to about 1/2 inch beyond rim. Fold up, and pinch so edge of pie is raised from rim.

Nutrition

199 calories; protein 2.4g; carbohydrates 17.9g; fat 13g; sodium 146.3mg.

Fried Apples

Servings:4

Ingredients

¼ cup vegetable oil
1 pinch salt
¼ cup maple flavored syrup
5 apples - peeled, cored and sliced

Directions

Melt oil or butter in a medium-sized cast iron pan over medium heat. Lay the apple slices in the oil or butter. Cook slowly, turning slices as they start to break down.

When they are soft on both sides, season with a pinch of salt and the syrup.

Nutrition

263 calories; protein 0.4g; carbohydrates 37.5g; fat 14.1g; sodium 13.7mg.

Fruit Trifle

Prep:15 mins
Additional:1 hr
Servings:12

Ingredients

1 (12 ounce) package frozen blueberries
2 (16 ounce) tubs reduced-fat frozen whipped topping, thawed
2 cups chopped fresh strawberries
1 (12 ounce) package frozen peach slices, chopped
1 (6 ounce) container fresh raspberries
1 prepared angel food cake, cut into chunks

Directions

Pour the blueberries into a strainer, rinse with water, and shake off excess water. Spread the berries out onto paper towels to dry slightly. In a deep, clear glass bowl or trifle bowl, spread a layer of angel food cake chunks. Scatter the cake with chopped strawberries in a thin layer. Sprinkle the strawberries with a layer of blueberries, followed by a layer of chopped peach slices. Sprinkle a few fresh raspberries over the peaches. Dollop a layer of whipped topping, then repeat layers until all cake and fruit has been used. Finish trifle with a layer of whipped topping. Cover the trifle, and refrigerate until chilled, about 1 hour.

Nutrition

295 calories; protein 2.3g; carbohydrates 55.1g; fat 8.9g; sodium 212mg.

Melon Popsicles

Prep time5 mins
Serves: 4 melon popsicles

Ingredients

3 cups chopped melon (honeydew, cantaloupe or watermelon)
1 teaspoon lime juice or lemon juice

Directions

Put the melon and lime or lemon juice in your blender and blend until very smooth.

Divide mixture between ice pop molds or 4 paper cups, leaving a little room at the top for expansion.

If using cups, place them in a baking dish for stability and insert a wooden stick in each cup.

Freeze for 30 minutes, and if using paper cups, straighten the sticks if they have moved off center.

Freeze for 1 more hour, or until solid.

Cocoa Fat Bombs

Prep:20 mins
Cook:12 mins
Additional:4 hrs 28 mins
Servings:72

Ingredients

1/2 cup nut butter of choice or coconut butter
1/4 cup cocoa or cacao powder
1/4 cup melted coconut oil
stevia to taste, or 1 tbsp liquid sweetener of choice
optional, I like to add 1/8 tsp salt

Directions

Stir all ingredients together until smooth. If too dry (depending on nut butter used), add additional coconut oil if needed. Pour into a small container, ice cube trays, candy molds, or this silicone mini cupcake tin. Freeze to set. Because coconut oil softens when warm, it's best to store these in the freezer.

Chocolate Chips Fudge

Prep:15 mins
Cook:2 hrs
Servings:28

Ingredients

2 cups semi-sweet chocolate chips
1 teaspoon vanilla extract
1 (14 ounce) can EAGLE BRAND® Sweetened Condensed Milk
1 cup peanut butter chips

Directions

In heavy saucepan, over low heat, melt chocolate chips and vanilla, stirring frequently.
Remove from heat. Add peanut butter chips; stir just to distribute chips throughout mixture.
Spread evenly into wax paper lined 8- or 9-inch square pan. Chill 2 hours or until firm. Turn fudge onto cutting board; peel off paper and cut into squares. Store leftovers covered in refrigerator.

Nutrition

172 calories; protein 2.9g; carbohydrates 16.3g; fat 7.5g; cholesterol 5mg; sodium 42.6mg.

Sugar Free Fudge

Prep:5 mins
Cook:11 mins
Additional:1 hr
Servings:16

Ingredients

3 cups granular sucralose sweetener (such as Splenda®)
¼ cup unsweetened cocoa powder
¼ cup peanut butter
¼ cup butter
1 cup evaporated milk

Directions

Line an 8-inch baking pan with aluminum foil. Clip a candy thermometer to the side of a saucepan.
1 cup evaporated milk
Combine sweetener, evaporated milk, and cocoa powder in the saucepan. Bring to a boil. Reduce heat to medium; cook and stir until the thermometer registers 234 degrees F or until a small amount of syrup dropped in cold water forms a soft ball, 5 to 10 minutes. Stir in peanut butter and butter until melted, about 1 minute.
Pour mixture into the prepared pan. Chill until set, 1 to 2 hours. Cut into squares.

Nutrition

76 calories; protein 2.4g; carbohydrates 4.4g; fat 6.3g; cholesterol 12.2mg; sodium 55.9mg.

Blueberry Granita

Prep:

15 mins

Additional:

4 hrs

Total:

4 hrs 15 mins

Servings:

4

Yield:

4 servings

Ingredients

2 ½ cups blueberries

½ cup white sugar

¾ cup water

1 tablespoon fresh lemon juice

Directions

1

Blend the blueberries and sugar in a food processor until smooth; strain through a fine-mesh strainer, pressing with a wooden spoon to separate the blueberry puree from any chunks of skin or seeds.

2

Stir the strained blueberry puree, water, and lemon juice together in a shallow glass baking dish or tray. Place the dish in the freezer; scrape and stir the blueberry mixture with a fork once an hour until evenly frozen and icy, about 4 hours. Scrape to fluff and lighten the ice crystals; spoon into chilled glasses to serve.

Nutritions

Per Serving: 149 calories; protein 0.7g; carbohydrates 38.5g; fat 0.3g; sodium 2.3mg.

Lemon Thins

Prep:

15 mins

Cook:

10 mins

Additional:

3 hrs 15 mins

Total:

3 hrs 40 mins

Servings:

24

Yield:

24 cookies

Ingredients

3 cups all-purpose flour
1 teaspoon baking powder
½ teaspoon baking soda
1 cup butter, softened
1 cup white sugar
⅓ cup lemon juice
Icing:
1 ¼ cups powdered sugar
2 tablespoons lemon juice

Directions

1

Sift flour, baking powder, and baking soda together in a large bowl.

2

Cream butter and sugar together in a bowl using an electric mixer until fluffy. Mix in lemon juice. Add flour mixture gradually, beating well after each addition.

3

Form dough into a log shape and wrap with waxed paper. Refrigerate for 3 to 4 hours.

4

Preheat the oven to 375 degrees F (190 degrees C). Line cookie sheets with parchment paper.

5

Slice chilled dough into roughly 1/8-inch slices. Place onto the prepared cookie sheets.

6

Bake in the preheated oven until edges are set and golden, 7 to 8 minutes. Remove from the oven and let cool completely, 15 to 30 minutes.

7

Combine powdered sugar and lemon juice in a bowl until smooth. Frost cooled cookies.

Nutritions
Per Serving: 184 calories; protein 1.7g; carbohydrates 27.2g; fat 7.8g; cholesterol 20.3mg; sodium 101.4mg.

Pepper Tapenade

Prep:

20 mins

Total:

20 mins

Servings:

8

Yield:

8 appetizer servings

Ingredients

1 cup sun-dried tomatoes, packed in oil, drained and oil reserved

⅓ cup reserved sun-dried tomato oil

3 tablespoons finely chopped red pepper

5 cloves garlic, finely chopped

6 ounces crumbled feta cheese

2 tablespoons dried basil

½ teaspoon ground black pepper

2 teaspoons balsamic vinegar

Directions

1

Finely chop sun-dried tomatoes and place in a large bowl. Stir in the reserved tomato oil, red pepper, garlic, feta cheese, dried basil, black pepper, and balsamic vinegar and mix well. Cover and chill for at least four hours before serving.

Nutritions

Per Serving: 173 calories; protein 4.1g; carbohydrates 5.5g; fat 15.6g; cholesterol 18.9mg; sodium 275mg.

Plum Sauce

Prep:

5 mins

Cook:

15 mins

Total:

20 mins

Servings:

10

Yield:

10 servings

Ingredients

¾ (16 ounce) jar plum jam

2 tablespoons vinegar

1 tablespoon brown sugar

1 tablespoon dried minced onion

1 teaspoon crushed red pepper flakes

1 clove garlic, minced

½ teaspoon ground ginger

Directions

1

In a saucepan over medium heat, combine jam, vinegar, brown sugar, dried onion, red pepper, garlic and ginger. Bring to a boil, stirring. Remove from heat.

Nutritions

Per Serving: 102 calories; protein 0.2g; carbohydrates 25.1g; fat 0.1g; sodium 11.4mg.

Falafel

Prep:

30 mins

Cook:

20 mins

Additional:

2 days

Total:

2 days

Servings:

6

Yield:

30 falafel

Ingredients

1 cup dried fava beans

water as needed

1 cup dried chickpeas

1 medium onion, coarsely chopped

2 cloves garlic, coarsely chopped

1 bunch flat-leaf parsley, leaves removed

1 pinch cayenne pepper

1 teaspoon ground coriander

¾ teaspoon ground cumin

1 teaspoon baking soda

1 pinch salt and freshly ground black pepper to taste

½ cup vegetable oil for frying, or as needed

Directions

1

Place fava beans in a bowl and cover with plenty of cold water. Soak for 2 days, changing the water daily (in hot weather change the water twice daily).

2

Soak chickpeas on the second day in a separate bowl in plenty of cold water.

3

Drain beans and chickpeas and rinse under cold running water; drain again. Remove the skins from the fava beans and discard them. Do not skip that   or the falafel will not taste good.

4

Combine fava beans, chickpeas, onion, garlic, and parsley leaves in the bowl of a food processor; pulse until pureed, scraping the sides often to ensure everything is evenly processed to a smooth paste. Add cayenne pepper, coriander, cumin, baking soda, salt, and pepper. Transfer to a bowl; cover and let mixture rest for 30 minutes.

5

Line a baking sheet or a large tray with waxed paper.

6

Shape the mixture into 25 to 30 evenly sized patties and place them on the prepared baking sheet, leaving at least 1/2 inch between them. Let rest, uncovered, for 30 minutes.

7

Preheat the oven to 350 degrees F (175 degrees C).

8

Pour oil into the bottom of a large skillet until it just covers the bottom. Heat until oil is hot enough to sizzle a breadcrumb.

9

Carefully lift the falafel from the waxed paper using a spatula. Fry a few falafel at a time and do not overcrowd the skillet. Fry until crisp and brown on the underside, 3 to 5 minutes. Flip, and fry on the other side until browned, another 3 to 5 minutes. Remove from skillet and transfer to a baking sheet. Place the finished falafel in the preheated oven to keep warm while you fry the rest, adding more oil to the pan as needed.

Lemon Cake

Prep:

20 mins

Cook:

45 mins

Additional:

1 hr 10 mins

Total:

2 hrs 15 mins

Servings:

12

Yield:

12 servings

Ingredients

10 tablespoons milk, divided

1 tablespoon dried lavender buds

1 ½ cups white sugar

½ cup butter, melted

5 eggs

¾ cup lemon juice, divided

1 ½ lemon, zested

2 cups cake flour

1 teaspoon baking powder

1 cup confectioners' sugar

Directions

1

Preheat oven to 325 degrees F (165 degrees C). Grease a fluted tube pan (such as Bundt®) generously.

2

Measure 5 tablespoons milk into a microwave-safe bowl. Heat in the microwave until warmed through, 30 to 45 seconds. Add lavender buds. Let steep to release their flavor, 10 to 15 minutes.

3

Whisk white sugar and butter together in a large bowl until creamy. Whisk in eggs, 1 at a time, whisking well after each addition. Add 1/2 cup lemon juice and lemon zest; mix until well-blended. Stir milk and lavender buds into the batter.

4

Sift cake flour and baking powder together in a bowl. Slowly fold into the batter, stirring well to prevent lumps. Pour into the greased tube pan.

5

Bake in the preheated oven until a toothpick inserted into the center of the cake comes out clean, 45 to 55 minutes. Cool in the pan for 5 minutes. Invert onto a wire rack to cool completely, at least 30 minutes.

6

Whisk remaining 5 tablespoons milk, 1/4 cup lemon juice, and confectioners' sugar together in a small bowl to make glaze; drizzle over the cooled cake. Let stand until glaze is set, about 30 minutes.

Nutritions
Per Serving: 329 calories; protein 4.8g; carbohydrates 56.3g; fat 10g; cholesterol 89.6mg; sodium 126.9mg.

CHAPTER 8: SMOOTHIES AND DRINKS

Ginger Tea

Prep:5 mins
Cook:10 mins
Additional:5 mins
Servings:1

Ingredients

8 ounces apple cider
1 (2 g) bag green tea
1 (2 inch) piece fresh ginger, peeled and sliced

Directions

Combine apple cider and ginger in a saucepan; bring to a boil. Boil for 2 to 3 minutes.
Place tea bag in a mug. Pour boiling cider into the mug, straining out the ginger slices. Steep for 1 to 2 minutes. Remove tea bag.

Nutrition

133 calories; protein 0.2g; carbohydrates 33.1g; fat 0.1g; sodium 27.4mg.

Grape Drink

Prep Time5 mins
Cook Time20 mins

Ingredients

For Grape Juice
300 grams grapes seedless
1/2 lemon
400 ml water
5 to 6 Ice Cubes
1/3 cup sugar
For Grape Soda
250 ml soda water
lemon wedge
½ sprig mint leaves

Directions

Making Grape Juice
Pour water into a saucepan.
Add seedless grapes and bring to a boil.
When the water starts to boil. Add sugar and mix well.
Add lemon juice to prevent the sugar from caramelizing.
Boil for 15 to 20 minutes and turn off the flame.
Leave until it cools down to room temperature.
Later make them into juice and transfer it into a clean & dry jar, store in the refrigerator.
Making Grape Soda
Take Ice Cubes into a glass.
Add ¼ cup Grape Juice.
Pour soda water.put a lemon wedge and a mint sprig and serve chilled.

Honey Cinnamon Latte

INGREDIENTS

FOR THE SIMPLE SYRUP:
¾ cup honey
1 ½ teaspoons vanilla extract
3 cinnamon sticks
¾ cup water
FOR SERVING:
ice cubes
cold brew coffee concentrate
whole milk or half and half*
sprinkle of ground cinnamon

DIRECTIONS

Add the water, honey and cinnamon sticks to a small saucepan. Set the pan over medium-high heat and cook, stirring frequently, until the honey has completely dissolved into the water. Let the mixture just come to a boil, then turn down the heat and let simmer gently for 5 minutes. Remove from the heat and stir in the vanilla extract.
Let the mixture cool completely then remove the cinnamon sticks (and discard).
Store the syrup in the refrigerator until ready to use.
TO SERVE:
Add some ice cubes to a serving glass. Pour in the cold brew coffee. Add in the desired amount of milk and honey cinnamon simple syrup, then mix to combine. Sprinkle the top with a touch of cinnamon. Serve immediately.

Aloe Vera Smoothie

PREP TIME5 mins
TOTAL TIME5 mins

INGREDIENTS

5 strawberries

1 cup almond milk

1 banana

½ cup ice

1 -2 oz aloe vera

Strawberry Milk Shake

Prep:25 mins
Cook:0 mins
Total:25 mins
Servings:2 servings

Ingredients

1/2 pound fresh strawberries
Small whole strawberries
1 tablespoon sugar
1 teaspoon vanilla extract
1 pint vanilla ice cream
1/2 cup milk

Directions

Gather the ingredients.

Cut the tops off the strawberries and slice them into a few pieces.

In a medium bowl, combine the sliced strawberries, sugar, and vanilla extract and stir to combine well.

Set aside and allow to sit for at least 20 minutes and for up to 1 hour.

Place the strawberries with any juices, ice cream, and milk in a blender. Blend until smooth.

Pour into large glasses and, if desired, put a strawberry on the rim of each glass.

Almond Milk

Prep:10 mins
Cook:3 mins
Servings:4

Ingredients

4 cups water, divided
¼ cup raw unsalted almonds
1 tablespoon tapioca flour
1 teaspoon soy lecithin
1 dash vanilla extract

Directions

Combine 1 cup water and tapioca flour in a microwave-safe cup; heat in microwave until boiling, about 4 minutes.
Combine tapioca mixture, remaining 3 cups water, almonds, soy lecithin, and vanilla extract in a high-powered blender; blend on high until smooth.
Strain mixture through cheese cloth layers into a container. Keep refrigerated.

Nutrition

68 calories; protein 1.9g; carbohydrates 3.5g; fat 5.6g; sodium 7.3mg

Beetrootroot ice

INGREDIENTS

ICE CREAM
200 g raw beetroot (about 2 medium beets – 100 ml freshly pressed beet juice)
300 ml (1 1/4 cup) heavy cream, 35-40% fat
finely grated zest from 1 lemon
2 tbsp. lemon juice
15 g fresh ginger
200 ml (3/4 cup + 1 1/2 tbsp.) milk, 3% fat
90 g (1/3 cup + 1 1/2 tbsp.) granulated sugar
1 tbsp. cornstarch
pinch of salt
1 tbsp. vodka (can be omitted)

DIRECTIONS

BEETROOT & GINGER ICE CREAM
Trim the edges of the beet roots. Peel them if they are very dirty, if not, washing them is enough. Cut them in smaller pieces and process them in a juicer together with the ginger. In a medium bowl, combine the beet juice, cream, lemon zest and juice.
In a small bowl, whisk together the cornstarch with 2 tbsp. of the milk. Heat the remaining milk, sugar and salt in a small saucepan until it comes almost to a boil and the sugar melts. Whisk in the cornstarch slurry and cook over low heat, stirring vigorously, until mixture thickens. Remove from the heat and mix with the beet juice and cream mixture. Stir until combined.
Let mixture cool completely. If you wish to speed things up a little, put the bowl in an ice bath and stir until cool. Cover the bowl with a lid or

plastic wrap and store in fridge until completely cold, preferably overnight.

Stir in vodka if using. Churn the ice cream in an ice cream maker according to your manufacturer's Directions.

Transfer ice cream to a freezer container. Smooth the top with a spatula, then loosely cover the surface of the ice cream with wax paper and freeze until almost solid, about 2-4 hours.

Pumpkin Spices Drink

Prep:10 mins
Total:10 mins
Servings:2

Ingredients

1 cup unsweetened almond milk
½ cup canned pumpkin
1 pinch ground ginger
2 bananas, sliced and frozen
1 scoop vanilla protein powder
½ teaspoon vanilla extract
2 dates, pitted
1 pinch ground cinnamon
1 pinch ground cloves

Directions

Blend almond milk, bananas, pumpkin, dates, protein powder, vanilla extract, nutmeg, cinnamon, cloves, and ginger together in a blender until smooth.

Nutrition

280 calories; protein 22g; carbohydrates 45.6g; fat 3g; cholesterol 6.3mg; sodium 191.8mg.

Baby Spinach and Dill Smoothie

Yield: 1

Ingredients

- ½ pear
- 1 cup frozen pineapple
- 1 cup chopped and seeded cucumber
- ¼ cup chopped fresh dill
- 1 cup baby spinach
- 1 small avocado
- 2 tablespoons lime juice
- 1-inch knob fresh gingerroot, peeled
- 3-4 ice cubes
- 1 tablespoon organic chia seeds

1 ¼ cup water

Directions

Place all ingredients, except for the ice and chia seeds, in a high speed blender and process until smooth and creamy. Add the ice and process again. Stir in chia seeds. Drink chilled.

Tofu and Berry Smoothie

Makes 1 serving (serving size: 2 cups)

Ingredients

1 cup frozen blueberries
1 tablespoon agave nectar or honey
1/2 cup pomegranate juice
1/2 cup crushed ice
1/2 cup (4 ounces) silken tofu

Directions

In a blender, combine ingredients; blend until smooth.

Nutrition

271 calories; fat 4.1g; saturated fat 0.5g; mono fat 0.7g; poly fat 2.2g; protein 7g; carbohydrates 56g; fiber 4g; iron 1mg; sodium 22mg; calcium 68mg.

SMOOTH SWEET TEA

Prep:5 mins
Cook:15 mins
Additional:3 hrs
Servings:8

Ingredients

1 pinch baking soda
¾ cup white sugar
6 tea bags
6 cups cool water
2 cups boiling water

Directions

Sprinkle a pinch of baking soda into a 64-ounce, heat-proof, glass pitcher. Pour in boiling water, and add tea bags. Cover, and allow to steep for 15 minutes.
Remove tea bags, and discard; stir in sugar until dissolved. Pour in cool water, then refrigerate until cold.

Nutrition

73 calories; carbohydrates 18.7g; sodium 41.3mg.

CPSIA information can be obtained
at www.ICGtesting.com
Printed in the USA
BVHW091356210621
610121BV00017B/453